Juice Boost!

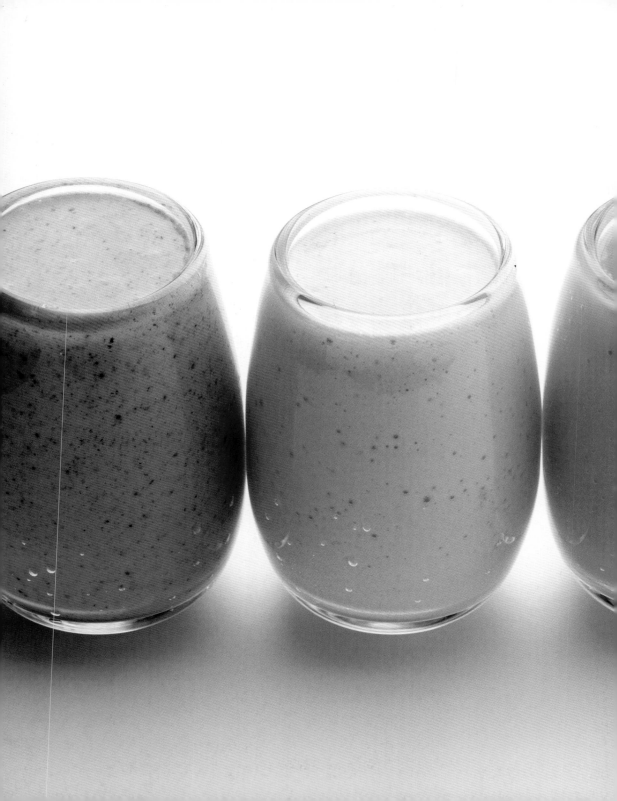

Juice Boost!

Juices, Smoothies & Boosters for Supercharged Health

DUNCAN BAIRD PUBLISHERS

LONDON

This book is dedicated to our incredibly hard-working team at Crussh juice bars in the UK. Each day our kitchen team, our store managers and our fantastic team members put their hearts and souls into making it happen at Crussh. To our head office team as well, without whom we wouldn't have the support needed to deliver great juices and smoothies every day to our fabulous customers!

 This book is a compilation of recipes collected from across the Crussh family, from the most experienced to the newest team member, to help you move toward a healthier and tastier lifestyle.

Christopher Fung, Managing Director of Crussh UK

Juice Boost!
Juices, Smoothies & Boosters
for Supercharged Health

Distributed in the USA and Canada by
Sterling Publishing Co., Inc.
387 Park Avenue South
New York, NY 10016-8810

First published in the UK and USA in 2013 by
Duncan Baird Publishers, an imprint of
Watkins Publishing Limited
Sixth Floor, 75 Wells Street
London W1T 3QH

A member of Osprey Group

ISBN: 978-1-84899-090-6

10 9 8 7 6 5 4 3 2 1

Crussh Mangaging Author: Christopher Fung
Managing Editor: Grace Cheetham
Editor: Wendy Hobson
Managing Designer: Manisha Patel
Designer & Commissioned artwork: Sailesh Patel
Production: Uzma Taj
Commissioned photography: William Lingwood
Food Stylist: Emily Jonzen
Prop Stylist: Lucy Harvey

Typeset in Segoe and Cocon
Color reproduction by XY Digital
Printed in China

For information about custom editions, special sales,
premium and corporate purchases, please contact
Sterling Special Sales Department at
800-805-5489 or specialsales@sterlingpub.com.

Publisher's note: While every care has been taken in compiling the recipes for this book, Watkins Publishing Limited, or any other persons who have been involved in working on this publication, cannot accept responsibility for any errors or omissions, inadvertent or not, that may be found in the recipes or text, nor for any problems that may arise as a result of preparing one of these recipes. If you are pregnant or breastfeeding or have any special dietary requirements or medical conditions, it is advisable to consult a medical professional before following any of the recipes contained in this book.

Notes on the Recipes
Unless otherwise stated:
Use medium fruit and vegetables
Use fresh ingredients, including herbs and chilies
1 tsp. = 5ml   1 tbsp. = 15ml   1 cup = 240ml

Contents

h

is for health

h is for health

This book is packed with all you need to know about making juicing a part of your happy and healthy lifestyle.

J

is for juices

j is for juices

Fresh fruit and vegetable juices are bursting with vital vitamins, minerals, phytochemicals and enzymes—the easy way to a total health makeover.

S

is for smoothies

s is for smoothies

Creamy-smooth drinks that are made from the whole fruit—including all the fiber—and often protein-rich yogurt or milk to get you ready for the day.

b

is for boosters

b is for boosters

An extra shot of goodness, such as ginseng, spirulina or aloe vera, can be added to either a juice or a smoothie for a real nutritional punch.

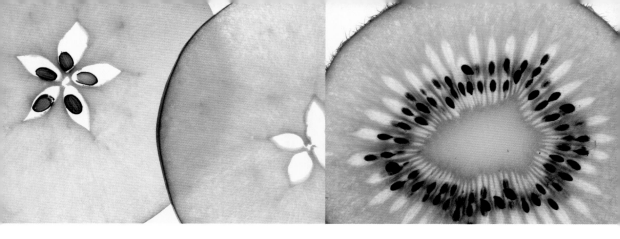

get ready for juicing

Welcome to feeling good, having more energy, looking slimmer and feeling healthier! Juicing can do all this for you—and more. So let us introduce you to the wonderful, healthy world of juicing—and you'll never look back.

Freshly pressed juices, smoothies and boosted juices are just packed with life-enhancing nutrients, ready and waiting for your body to absorb in an instant. There's no comparison even with the "freshly squeezed" juices in the supermarket, because your juices are only seconds old, so they haven't lost any of those high-powered nutrients that are so vital to your health and well-being.

Plus there are no extra sweeteners,

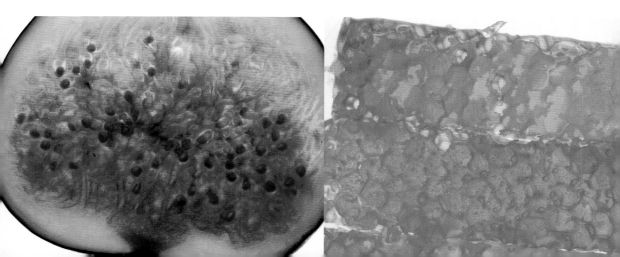

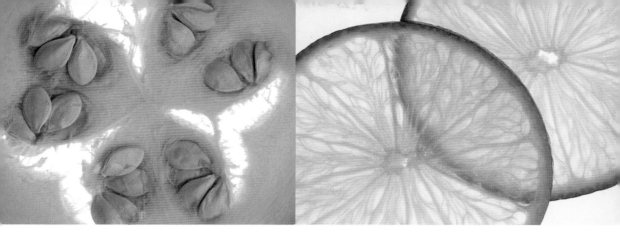

additives or preservatives to taint the purity of your juices. They are just the natural goodness and nothing else.

All the essential information you need to find out about these fabulous, life-enhancing foods-in-a-glass is included in this book—from the low-down on just how good they are, to the high-impact recipes themselves.

Full of flavor, packed with nutrients and bringing you all the colors of the rainbow, you'll soon clue into the fruits and vegetables that give you the boost you are looking for—fitness, energy or simply all-round good health. So the sooner you start juicing, the quicker you'll be looking good and feeling great!

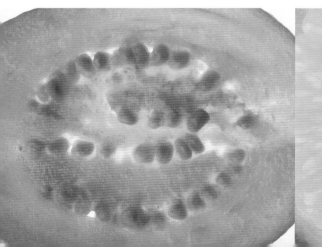

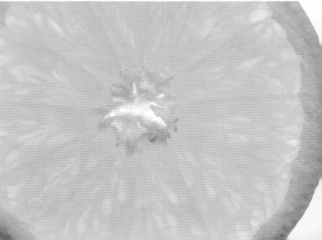

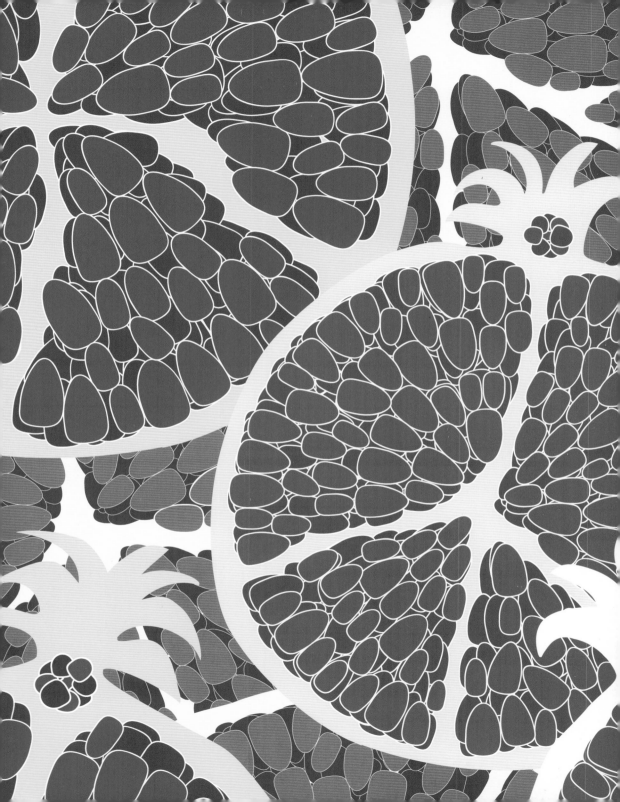

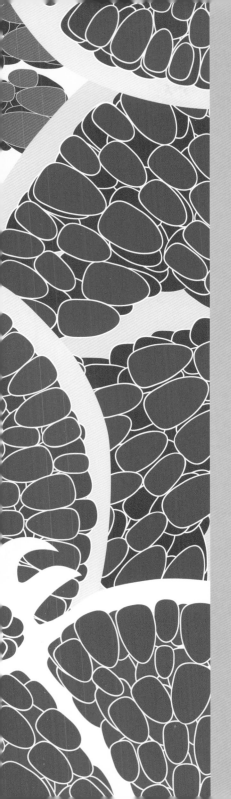

h

is for health

If you're looking for an instant **boost** to your health and well-being, start juicing now and you'll never look back. The **simplest** way to boost your diet with the **essential** nutrients you need, it will help you feel good, look great and surprise everyone with your new stores of **energy**.

It's all about getting the best out of **fresh** fruits and vegetables—extracting their nutritional essence—so that we can absorb all that **goodness** and rush it to where our bodies need it most. So let's not hang around—**let's get juicing!**

what is so great about juicing?

Looking for a burst of high-impact nutrients to get you performing to the max? Look no further.

Rushing around, cramming work, socializing, workouts, kids and whatever else into our diaries, the time for thinking about how we fuel all this activity is pretty limited. We eat fruit and veg, strive for the right balance of proteins and unrefined carbs, minimize the sugar and watch the fats.

But if we add freshly made juices to that mix, we get so much more.

Cooking any foods destroys some of their nutritional value, so juicing raw fruit and vegetables gives us a head start to healthy eating. Crucial enzymes that are responsible for the absorption of foods rarely survive the cooking process. But they thrive in the juicing process!

Juice fresh fruits and vegetables and you instantly release the valuable nutrients crammed inside: not just enzymes but vitamins, minerals, antioxidants and trace elements. And because they have already been released from the fibrous membranes of the vegetable or fruit, they are ready for your body to absorb without using more time and energy to digest them. Take beta-carotene,

for example. You get about 1% of that immune-boosting nutrient if you eat a carrot. And if you juice it? An amazing 100%.

As well as hanging onto all the nutrients, juice doesn't waste the valuable water content, an essential to life itself. Our brain is 80% water, and we all know how vital it is to keep our brains—as well as the rest of our bodies—properly hydrated.

And the busier we are, the less time we want to spend on food preparation. So how do you prepare fruit and veg for juicing? Wash them, get rid of any large pits or thick skins ... and that's it!

Of course, we could avoid any prep at all by taking supplements. But it is a proven fact that it is far better to obtain nutrients from food than from a jar—besides where's the fun in that? The flavors, the textures and the wonderful variety of fruit and vegetable combos you can create in your own kitchen make juicing such an enjoyable part of your day.

It's so easy to make juicing part of your healthy eating plan, and you'll feel the benefits so quickly, the only thing you are likely to regret is not having started sooner.

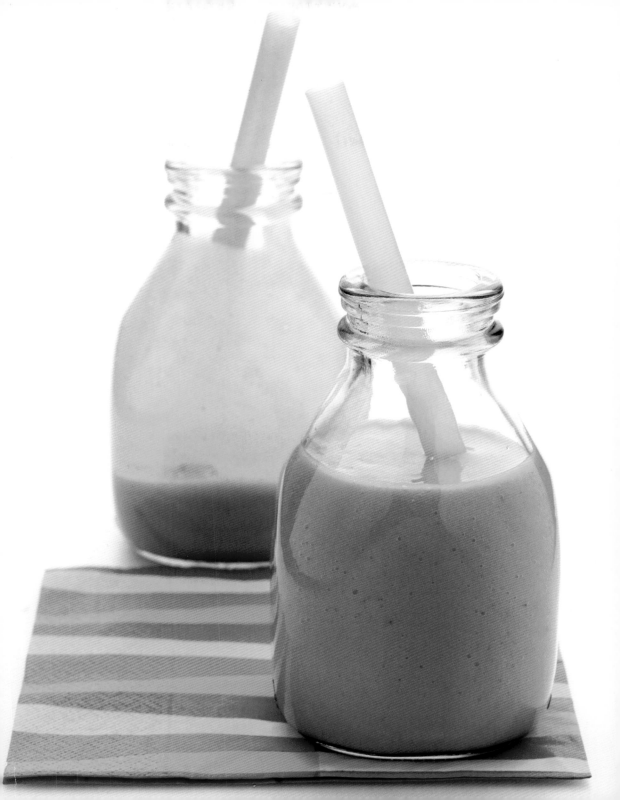

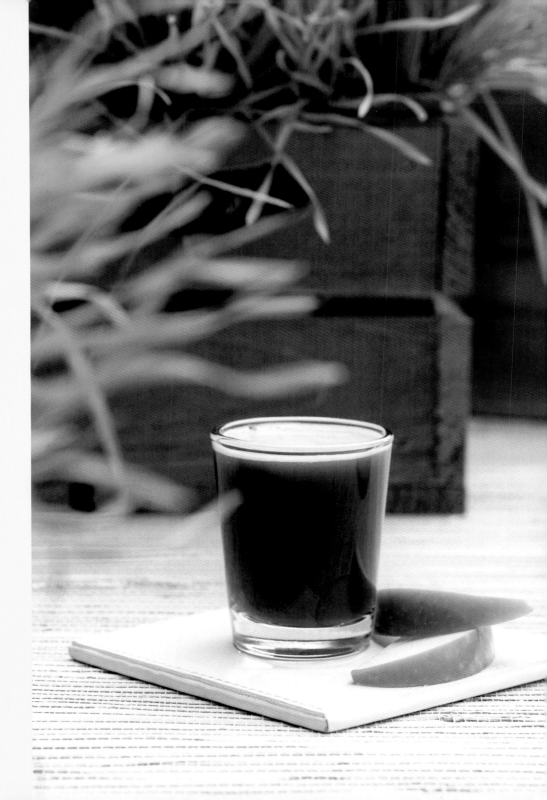

what can juicing do for you?

To stay fit and healthy, your body doesn't just need a balanced diet of protein, complex carbohydrates and fats. It's essential to get the required amounts of vitamins, minerals and trace elements. Required only in tiny quantities, they have a disproportionate effect on how well your body functions, so ultimately your good health relies on them.

Run short of folic acid and your hair and nails will suffer. If you don't have the antioxidants your body needs, it will affect the tone and suppleness of your skin. Without the right balance of vitamins and minerals, your metabolism will not run efficiently, you could lack energy, impair your immune system, or open yourself up to all kinds of illnesses and health problems, from the insignificant to the more serious.

And where do free radicals fit into all this? Those rampaging particles we've heard about damage our cell structure, causing those dreaded signs of aging: wrinkles, sagging skin, loss of muscle tone and lack of energy. Highly reactive molecules with one unpaired electron, free radicals range through the body, attacking and stealing the electrons from healthy cells to make themselves stable. This sets up a chain reaction, releasing new free radicals to wreak their havoc. The solution is to include enough antioxidants in our diet to combat that damage, and where better to find them than in fresh fruit and vegetable juices.

Then there's the fact that some of us would like to shed a few pounds. We know we shouldn't turn to the quick fix of fat- and sugar-laden junk food. But when we are hungry and in a rush, munching on a bag of carrots doesn't seem that appealing. Convert them to juice, however, and you have a super-nutritious boost in an easily assimilated form that is fresh, delicious and satisfying. So juicing can be a route back to healthy eating to maintain a healthy weight.

about juicers

To make our juices, all you need is a juicer—which separates the juice from the pulp—and a blender—which chops everything to a puree.

Check out the different juicers on the market—maybe borrow one for a few days—before you decide which one is right for you. The price range is wide because they vary from basic to high-tech. But if your juicer is not effective and convenient you are likely to give up, so buy the best you can.

There are two main kinds of juicer. (There's also hydraulic juicers—but you'll only see them at juice bars.)

Centrifugal juicers These have a spinning grater that extracts the juice from the pulp. Although cheaper, you have to feed in the fruit and veg in smaller pieces and the juice has slightly lower nutrient levels.

Masticating juicers These are the big guys. They liquidize the fruit and veg, then ram it through a fine mesh. They are more expensive, but more powerful with higher nutrient yields.

Whichever juicer you choose, go for a reputable manufacturer and check that it's easy to clean, and whether any parts can go in the dishwasher.

Use juicers for Hard fruits and most vegetables, such as apples, beets, carrots, celery, kale, spinach.

about blenders & squeezers

You probably already have a blender or food processor in the kitchen. Use them when you are making smoothies to get a rich, creamy finish, and also for the second phase of making juices in which hard vegetables are combined with soft fruits.

Any blender or food processor will do. If you don't have one, you can even make smoothies with an immersion blender, which can be used in a bowl or pan. Most of us already have one of these and, if not, they are cheap to buy.

Use blenders for Soft fruits and vegetables, such as avocados, bananas, blackberries, blackcurrants, blueberries, cranberries, dates, kiwis, lychees, mangoes, passionfruit, peaches, raspberries, strawberries.

Where the recipes include citrus juices, such as orange juice, these should be freshly pressed through a citrus squeezer. You can use any kind, from a simple, conical squeezer that you press the orange half onto, or one that comes as part of your food processor. If you only need a small quantity of juice—say a squeeze of lime juice to zing up the flavors—then a small hand squeezer works well.

Use squeezers for Citrus fruits, such as lemons, limes, oranges.

how it's done

Prepare your juice or smoothie when you want to drink it so it's as fresh and nutritious as it can be.

First, choose your fruit and veg. It's always best to use fresh, seasonal produce where possible—organic is also preferable. Ripe fruit makes for a tastier and more colorful juice. Scrub off any dirt, wash the fruit or veg in warm water, then rinse. We like to use organic vegetable wash.

Remove any large pits or tough skins, but small seeds and thinner skins are fine. Cut, or preferably tear, the fruit and veg into pieces that will fit into your juicer. Then, just juice!

Over the years we have developed our view of what makes a great smoothie! We believe our smoothies are the best in the world, with the right balance of thickness and containing more fruit than those you'll find at any juice or smoothie bar. We are purists in that our smoothies contain only fruit, yogurt and 100% juice. There's no ice in our smoothies and we use low-fat, frozen probiotic yogurt.

When you make our recipes at home, you'll get the best, thickest smoothies if you freeze your soft fruits overnight. This way you get the full intensity of flavor from the fruit without having to dilute it with ice cubes to cool it down.

We also recommend freezing your yogurt to get that thick, creamy texture you want in your smoothie.

Of course, sometimes you want the instant gratification of making your smoothie right away. It will still taste great if you go ahead without freezing the ingredients. But you may want to keep some fruit in the freezer ready for a quick smoothie any time.

Another tip for quick smoothies is to use 100% fresh juices from the chilled display in your supermarket. This saves you having to get the juicer out and you're going straight in with the blender to make your perfect smoothie. Trying out different juices as your base will open up new flavor combinations—if you keep the citrus and tropical fruit juices together (orange, pineapple, mango, and so on) and more neutral juices together (like apple and grape), you won't go wrong when you create great new smoothies.

Where we have used milk or soy milk, feel free to experiment with the wide range of dairy-free alternatives becoming increasingly available from good supermarkets, such as almond, hazelnut, oat and rice milks. They are all great options.

how to use
this book

Every one of these recipes is packed
with super-nutrients that will give you
a health boost. The recipes are divided
into three sections.

J is for juices In this chapter,
you'll find juices made from fruits,
vegetables or a delicious combination
of both. Some are made just by juicing
the ingredients in a juicer. Some
include freshly squeezed citrus juice.
Others are juiced and then blended
to make the most of hard fruits and
vegetables and also soft fruits. And
don't forget the juicers' favorite:
wheatgrass.

S is for smoothies The next
chapter concentrates on the blender,
liquidizing fruits and vegetables, milk,
yogurt, spices and herbs to create a
range of deliciously creamy, healthy
smoothies—perfect for breakfast,
lunch or a mid-afternoon boost.

B is for boosters Finally, we will
introduce you to super-charged
juicing! With extra boosts of
supplements or powerfoods, such
as coenzyme Q10, ginseng, chia seeds
and aloe vera, these babies really pack
a nutritional punch.

Juicing should be fun, so don't get
too hung up on quantities—just start
juicing. A healthier body and a sharper
mind are waiting!

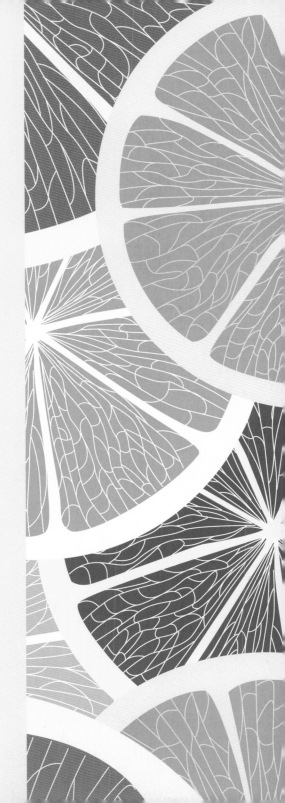

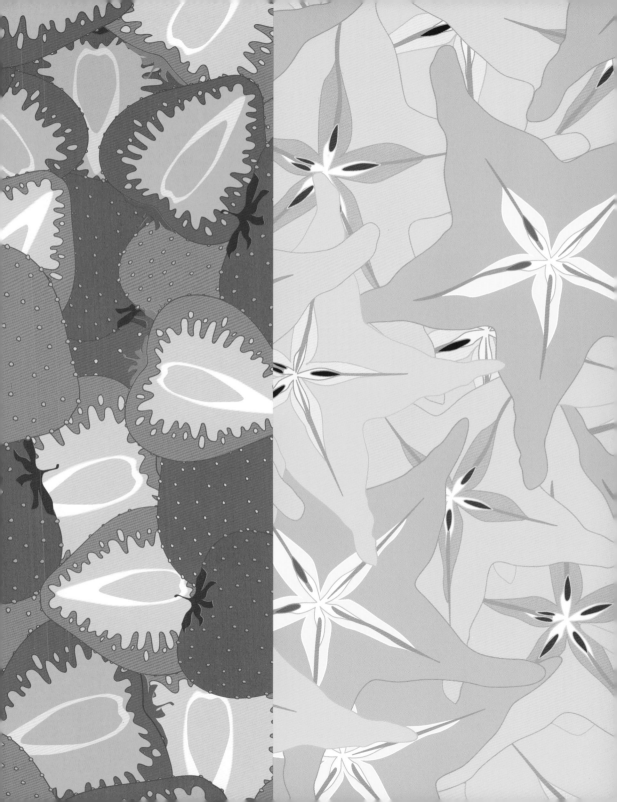

finding out about nutrients

Every juice in this book is packed with super-goodness. And every delicious recipe tells you just which valuable nutrients it contains.

Packed with Nutrients listed under this heading provide at least 20% of the daily amount of the nutrient recommended by the Food and Nutrition Board. But it may be as much as 100%—or even more.

Plenty of This shows that the juice provides 10–20% of the recommended daily intake of those nutrients listed under this heading.

Also contains This tells you any other nutrients that are present in smaller quantities, less than 10% of the recommended allowance.

They are listed in standard order:
Vitamins The familiar vitamins, essential for good health.
Minerals Major minerals, like calcium, magnesium and iron.

Macronutrients Important dietary elements, like fiber, which you'll get in smoothies and blended juices.
Antioxidants, phytonutrients and trace elements Minute quantities of some elements make a big difference to our body function. Antioxidants, for example, are the molecules that fight cell-destroying free radicals. Exciting new research is showing how flavonoids and ellagic acid could help our bodies fend off chronic diseases.

Detoxing with juicing

When you start juicing, you may notice that you need to go to the bathroom more often or you may experience a slight headache, which should pass in a few days. This is the result of your body getting rid of toxins and preparing to get back to full health. If symptoms persist, consult your medical practitioner.

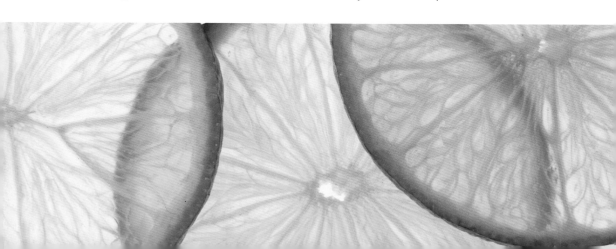

follow the juice rainbow

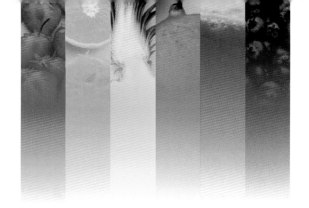

The color of each fruit gives you a clue as to the nutrients it contains, so you can follow the colors of the juicing rainbow to find the nutrients you are looking for.

Follow the red rainbow ...
Red fruits and vegetables contain antioxidants that chase down and destroy harmful free radicals in our bodies. They can help keep your blood pressure on an even keel, lower harmful cholesterol and protect you against the signs of aging ... they may even help reduce the risk of some cancers.

Follow the orange rainbow ...
And you'll find your way to immune-boosting country. For protection from all the bad stuff that life throws at us, for a healthy heart and great-looking skin and hair, orange is best.

Follow the yellow rainbow ...
This is the road to looking good and staying young—in body and mind. Yellow fruits and veg are the ones that can help maintain healthy bones and supple joints. Not to mention playing their part to battle the harmful free radicals that contribute to aging.

Follow the green rainbow ...
Some of the green top-of-the-range superfoods—like spinach and kale—are crammed with health-giving nutrients that are great for a healthy digestive system, to keep cholesterol in check, boost your immune system and lower blood pressure. Green is clearly the color for go!

Follow the purple rainbow ...
Supporting top-to-toe health, in this group you'll discover nutrients to boost your brain function—and who doesn't want to be smarter?—help control damaging cholesterol, boost your immune system and encourage your body to utilize nutrients efficiently.

Follow the white rainbow ...
When the spectrum comes together, all those big hitters are punching their weight on your side. With nutrients that activate your body's own defense system, they can help give your body a natural detox.

superfoods: fruit

Here is your at-a-glance guide to the nutrient
boost you can get from the fresh fruits
used in our juices, smoothies and boosted
juices—grouped into vitamins; minerals;
macronutrients; phytonutrients and trace
elements—and the health benefits, too.

FRUIT	PACKED WITH	WHAT'S IN IT FOR ME?
Apples	Beta-carotene; flavonoids	Can bring down your blood pressure and calm inflammation
Apricots	Beta-carotene; iron, potassium	Great for healthy eyes, skin and hair
Avocados	Vitamins B complex, C; potassium	Good for your heart health and lower cholesterol
Bananas	Potassium	Perfect for a boost of slow-release energy, good for the nerves and to help you keep your blood pressure level
Blackberries	Vitamins C, E, folic acid	Good for immune-system protection, they can also relieve inflammation
Blackcurrants	Vitamin C; flavonoids	Give your memory a boost—and who doesn't need that?—and a shot in the arm for the immune system
Blueberries	Vitamin C; flavonoids	Brilliant brain food—with a super-boost of nutrients
Cherries	Copper, manganese, potassium, zinc; antioxidants, flavonoids	Anti-inflammatory, so look for a soothing effect on the nerves, and they promote a healthy heart

FRUIT	PACKED WITH	WHAT'S IN IT FOR ME?
Chilies	Beta-carotene; flavonoids	Great for healthy skin—from the inside out—and to keep your blood pressure where it should be
Coconuts	Phosphate, potassium	For energy and strong bones
Cranberries	Vitamin C, beta-carotene; manganese; fiber	News is that they help to prevent urinary tract infections as well as supporting a healthy cardiovascular system
Cucumbers	Vitamin B complex	There's an energy boost here—and they can help you keep your hair looking great
Dates	Vitamins A, beta-carotene; iron, potassium; fiber	Good news for both your digestive and respiratory systems
Grapefruit	Vitamin C; flavonoids	Apart from the vitamin C boost, they can help regulate blood sugar levels and appetite
Grapes	Vitamins A, C, B6, folic acid; potassium	Can help you maintain a healthy heart and effective digestive system—plus there's an anti-aging bonus
Guavas	Vitamins A, B complex, C; potassium	Protect against some cancers, and are also good for a healthy heart
Kiwis	Vitamin C; fiber	Keep your vital immune system in good shape and sharpen your eyesight
Lemons	Vitamin C; limonene	Stave off those coughs and sneezes
Limes	Vitamin C; limonene	Another hit against infection, and they are good for healthy teeth and gums
Longan fruits	Vitamin C; copper, potassium	Great for the circulation system

FRUIT	PACKED WITH	WHAT'S IN IT FOR ME?
Lychees	Vitamins B complex, C; copper, potassium; antioxidants; fiber	More good news for the circulation here, and they can also even out problems in the digestive system
Mangoes	Vitamins B complex, C, E, beta-carotene; fiber	All about the stomach—they ease problems and can prevent constipation
Mangosteens	Vitamins B complex, C; potassium	Antioxidants help resist infections and fight damaging free radicals, control heart rate and blood pressure
Melons, honeydew	Vitamin C, beta-carotene	For clear skin and shining eyes (but not a wet nose!)
Oranges	Vitamin C; flavonoids; limonene	All kinds of benefits, starting with supporting the immune system and helping fight infection, all the way to raising depleted blood sugar levels
Papayas	Vitamins B complex, C, beta-carotene; potassium	Good for skin and bones, with an added energy boost
Peaches	Vitamin C, beta-carotene; fiber	Perfect for those who exercise, they ease muscle weakness and relieve fatigue
Pears	Vitamin C; potassium	Cut that blood pressure back to normal and protect against free radical damage
Pears, Asian	Fiber	Good for the digestive system
Pineapples	Vitamin C; copper, manganese; fiber	Help your body to repair and restore
Plums	Vitamin E; potassium; flavonoids	Inhibit free radicals to reduce the signs of aging

FRUIT	PACKED WITH	WHAT'S IN IT FOR ME?
Pomegranates	Vitamin C; ellagic acid, flavonoids	Promote heart health and may reduce the risk of some cancers
Prunes	Vitamin B6; iron, potassium; fiber	Have anti-aging properties, promote healthy digestion and boost energy
Rambutans	Vitamin C; antioxidants, flavonoids	Watch out, germs, this is an immune-system boost
Raspberries	Vitamin C; ellagic acid, flavonoids	Soothing all the way—whether for pain or an irritable digestive tract
Redcurrants	Vitamin C; potassium; flavonoids	You'll soon see these are good to sharpen the brain—and they help maintain healthy eyesight too!
Starfruits	Vitamin C; flavonoids; fiber	Brain boosting and good for the immune system
Strawberries	Vitamin C; ellagic acid, flavonoids	Delicious summer favorites—and packed with nutrients to combat aching joints and improve brain function—win, win!
Tomatoes	Vitamins C, E, beta-carotene; potassium; fiber	Healthy skin, strong bones, plus an immune-system boost
Watermelons	Vitamins B1, B6, C	Balance your body's water in order to use fluid effectively and help soothe body tissues

superfoods: vegetables

Find out the great things these vegetables can do to boost your system, making you look and feel fitter and healthier. Nutrients are grouped into vitamins; minerals; macronutrients; phytonutrients and trace elements. What's in it for me tells you just some of the health benefits you can expect.

VEGETABLE	PACKED WITH	WHAT'S IN IT FOR ME?
Asparagus	Vitamins C, E, beta-carotene, folic acid; phosphate; fiber	Both a tonic and a sedative, asparagus can be a calming influence for those suffering from nervous problems
Beets	Vitamin C, folic acid; iron, potassium; flavonoids	Beets are a real superfood—they are even the choice of Paralympic champions—so try them if you want to work to become fitter, faster, stronger!
Carrots	Vitamins A, B complex, beta-carotene	The nutrients in carrots really do promote healthy eyes—and also control heart rate and blood pressure, and minimize those dreaded signs of aging
Celery	Potassium; fiber	Flushing out excess CO_2 and reducing unwanted acidity are among the benefits here
Fennel	Vitamins A, C, E; copper; antioxidants; fiber	So obviously soothing, this is the ultimate digestive aid, so add fennel to your juices if you have an unsettled system
Kale	Vitamin K, beta-carotene, folic acid; calcium, iron, magnesium	Essential for maintaining healthy skin, as well as encouraging bone strength and healthy circulation; it may also lower cholesterol—can't be bad!

VEGETABLE	PACKED WITH	WHAT'S IN IT FOR ME?
Pumpkins	Vitamins A, B complex; flavonoids	Apart from offering a range of valuable vitamins and antioxidants, the latest research also suggests an anti-cancer factor here
Spinach	Vitamins B6, K; calcium, iron, magnesium, potassium	Great for all aspects of health, the nutrients in spinach can protect against free radicals, help normalize heart rate and blood pressure, and are good for strong bones
Watercress	Vitamins C, K	High in antioxidants, let the valuable nutrients in your watercress juice wash over your brain to keep it spring cleaned
Wheatgrass	Vitamins A, C, E, B12; iron, calcium, potassium	An all-round superfood, wheatgrass will boost your metabolism and get you bouncing with energy— why not grow your own?
Zucchini	Vitamins C, beta-carotene, folic acid	Skin protection is a primary benefit, plus they help prevent anemia

superfoods: boosters & other ingredients

Flavor and health-promoting properties are added to our juices with these ingredients.

FOOD	WHAT'S IN IT FOR ME?
Acai berries	Anti-aging, anti-inflammatory and anti-cancer
Agave syrup	A sweet nectar—the perfectly natural sweetener
Aloe vera	In juices, it's anti-inflammatory and soothes the digestive system
Bee pollen	Protects against the signs of aging and is anti-inflammatory
Cacao nibs	An energy booster to invigorate and refresh
Cardamom	A great digestive that freshens the breath at the same time
Chia seeds	Newly promoted in the West, they offer all-round health benefits
Cinnamon	Sprinkle on your juices to ward off those winter colds
Coenzyme Q10	An effective brain booster to keep you sharp
Echinacea	Support your natural defenses
Ginger root	Soothe tired muscles, reduce inflammation—and it will aid your digestion, too
Ginkgo biloba	A boost to your mental energy
Ginseng	A great all-rounder, it can help reduce stress, flush toxins out of your body and boost energy levels
Goji berries	Cellulite busting and good for the reproductive system

FOOD	WHAT'S IN IT FOR ME?
Granola	Fiber, nutritious nuts and oats to keep you feeling satisfied
Guarana	A herb native to Brazil yields this refreshing tonic
Honey	Soothe sore throats and attack hay fever with a daily spoonful of local honey
Maple syrup	A wholesome and delicious natural sweetener with its own distinctive flavor
Mint	A fresh fragrance, great for the digestion, which can relieve headaches, too
Oats	An effective form of slow-release energy, they also help to lower cholesterol
Omega oil	Bringing you a healthy heart and flexible joints
Protein powder	A muscle-building booster
Pumpkin seeds	Give you flexible joints and good circulation to help you do your circuits
Spirulina	Loaded with anti-aging properties, promotes healthy nerves and tissues
Sunflower seeds	High in fiber, vitamins and minerals, these provide a healthy snack and an all-round health benefit in your juicing
Thai basil leaves	Both a natural tranquilizer and a refreshing nerve tonic
Tofu	Fights against cholesterol and works to mitigate the signs of aging
Vitamin B5	Alleviates stress by helping maintain an adequate supply of hormones
Vitamin C	Essential for good health, with particular attention to the respiratory system
Walnuts	Benefits to your blood pressure can be found here, as well as some great anti-aging properties
Wheat germ	High in fiber, the heart of the wheat
Yogurt	Helps build strong bones and teeth, plus it promotes the maintenance of healthy bacteria in the gut

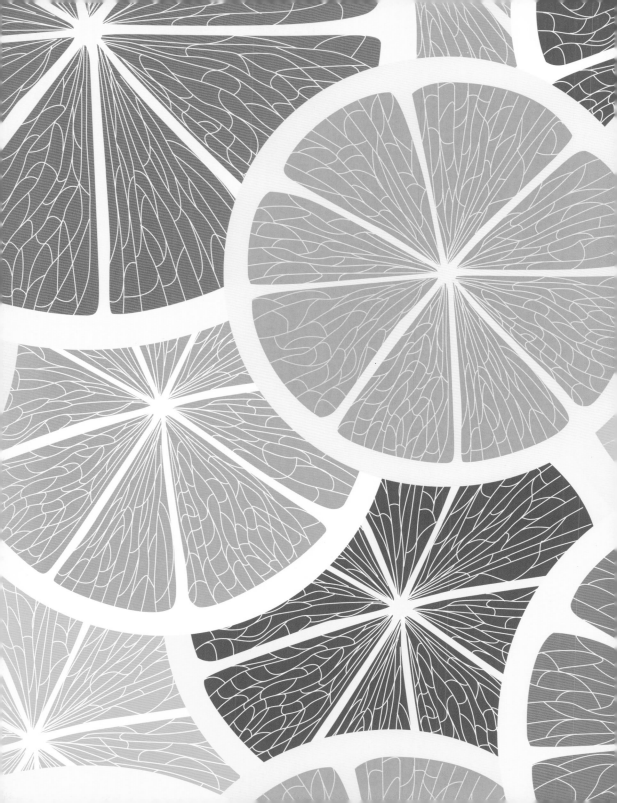

j

is for juices

Once you start on the adventure of making a **fresh juice** every day, you'll be hooked. This will be one of the **easiest** things you can do to transform your **health** and happiness. You'll feel the **benefits** pretty much immediately—you'll probably feel full of **energy** and **revitalized**, have a smoother, brighter complexion, and you're pretty sure to lose excess **weight**. Here you'll find a fantastic variety of juiced fruits to start you on your journey. And you can also discover the celebrity **beauty secret** of vegetable and fruit juice combinations.

When you pick
a papaya ...

Did you know?
Papaya is a natural tummy soother.
Its enzymes work wonders
for heartburn and
indigestion.

papaya love

Naturally sweet and beautifully bright,
you'll love waking up to this sunshine-filled
juice blend.

¼ papaya, peeled and seeded
5 oranges, halved
½ mango, peeled and pitted

How to do it Put the papaya through
an electric juicer. Squeeze the juice from the
oranges. (Alternatively, add ⅔ cup orange juice
instead of squeezing the oranges.) Pour the
juices into a blender or food processor, add the
mango and blend until smooth and creamy.
Serve immediately.

NUTRIENTS:
Packed with: vitamins
B6, C, beta-carotene;
magnesium, manganese,
phosphate, potassium
Plenty of: vitamins B1,
B2, B5, B7, folic acid;
copper, iron; fiber
Also contains: vitamins
B3, E; calcium, zinc;
flavonoids; limonene

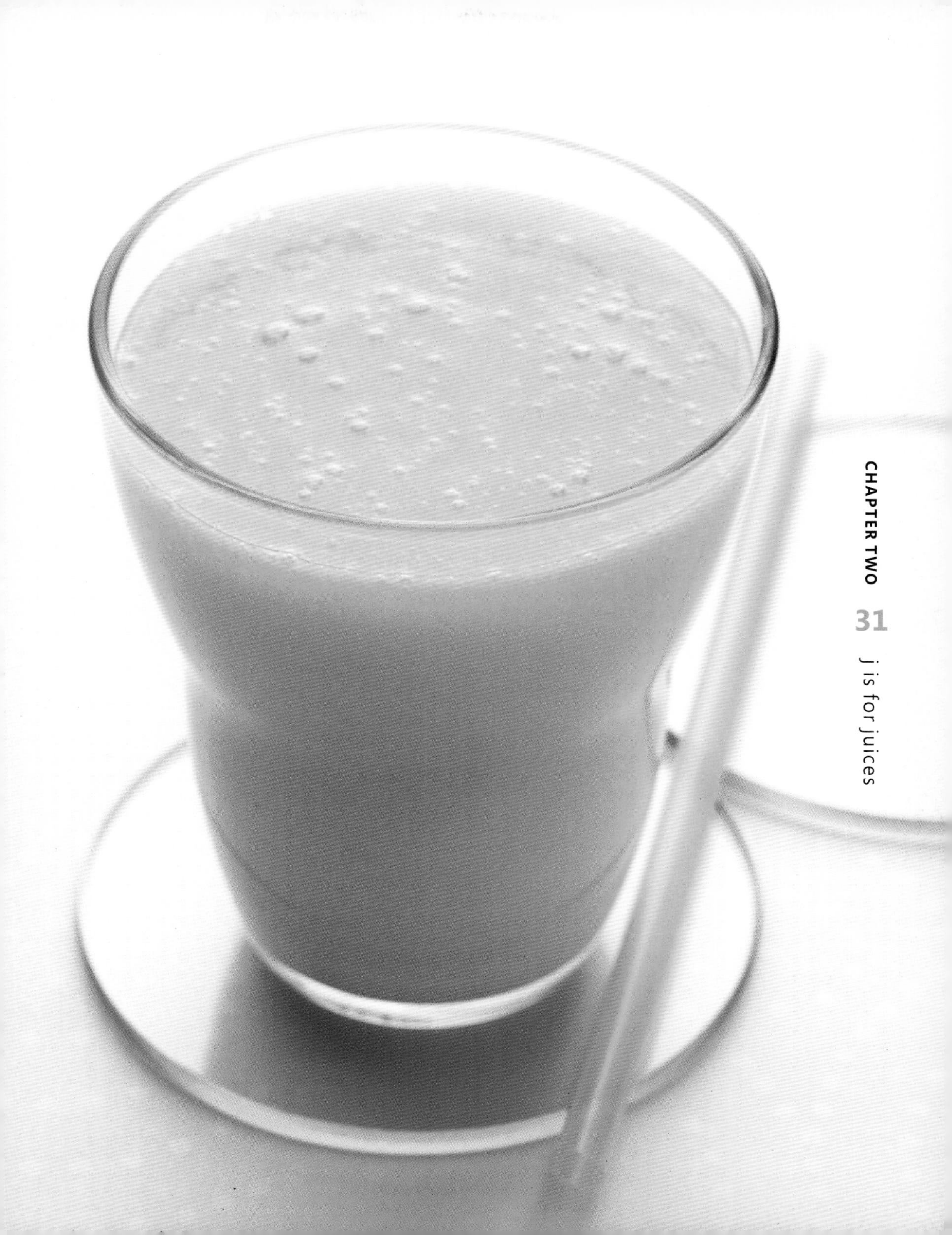

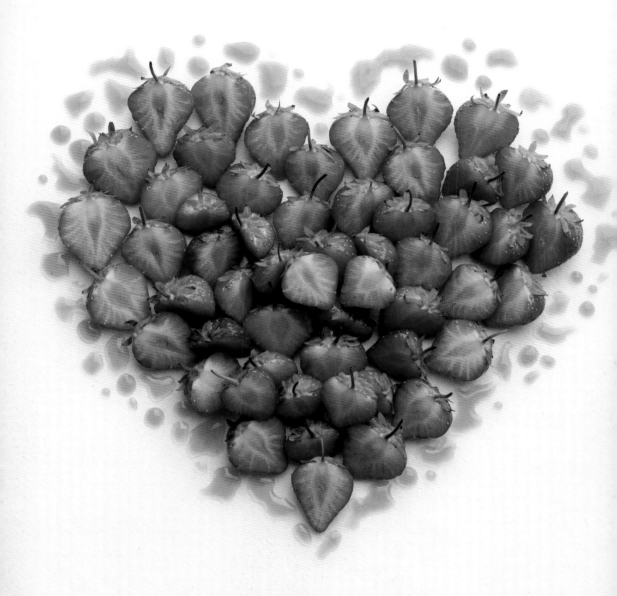

Say it with strawberries

love juice

Also known as Orange & Strawberry Sunrise, this classic drink is made with banana to make it rich and creamy, and with the great taste of fresh strawberries and peaches. This will bring a smile to any breakfast in bed!

4 oranges, halved
10 strawberries
1 banana
½ peach, pitted

How to do it Squeeze the juice from the oranges. (Alternatively, add ⅔ cup orange juice instead of squeezing the oranges.) Pour the juice into a blender or food processor, add all the remaining ingredients and blend until smooth and creamy. Serve immediately.

NUTRIENTS:
Packed with: vitamins B1, B5, B6, B7, C, beta-carotene, folic acid; magnesium, manganese, potassium
Plenty of: vitamins B2, B3; copper, iron, phosphate
Also contains: vitamin E; calcium, iodine, zinc; fiber; ellagic acid, flavonoids; limonene

enzyme digester

Give your digestive system a makeover with the soothing qualities of papaya and fragrant kiwi.

½ pineapple, peeled and cut into chunks
¼ papaya, peeled and seeded
1 kiwi, peeled and halved

How to do it Put all the ingredients through an electric juicer. Stir the juices together and serve immediately.

NUTRIENTS:
Packed with: vitamins C, beta-carotene; iron, magnesium, manganese, phosphate
Plenty of: vitamins B1, B5, B6; potassium, copper, zinc; fiber
Also contains: vitamins B2, B3, folic acid; calcium

rise & shine

This is one of our favorites as the weather gets warmer and the days brighter. Blood oranges come into season in the spring and the fresh tropical flavors of mango and passionfruit can't help but give you a lift in the morning!

2 pieces (about 2-inch cubes) peeled pineapple
3 blood oranges, halved
½ mango, peeled and pitted
½ passionfruit, pulp scooped out

How to do it Put the pineapple through an electric juicer. Squeeze the juice from the oranges. (Alternatively, add ⅔ cup orange juice instead of squeezing the oranges.) Pour the juices into a blender or food processor, add the mango and the passionfruit seeds and blend until smooth and creamy. Serve immediately.

NUTRIENTS:
Packed with: vitamins B6, C, beta-carotene; manganese, potassium;
Plenty of: vitamins B1, B2, B3, B5, B7, folic acid; calcium, copper, iron, magnesium, phosphate; fiber
Also contains: vitamin E; flavonoids, limonene

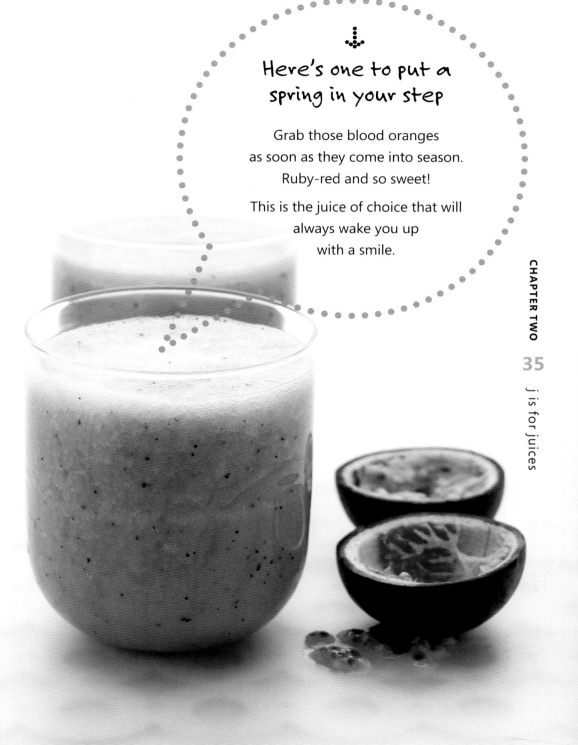

Here's one to put a spring in your step

Grab those blood oranges
as soon as they come into season.
Ruby-red and so sweet!

This is the juice of choice that will
always wake you up
with a smile.

simple morning juice

Just what you need in the morning to boost your energy levels while soothing your digestive system.

4 oranges, halved
1½ cups raspberries

How to do it Squeeze the juice from the oranges. Pour the juice into a blender or food processor, add the raspberries and blend until smooth. Serve immediately.

NUTRIENTS:
Packed with: vitamin C; manganese
Plenty of: vitamins B1, B6, B7, folic acid; potassium
Also contains: vitamins B2, B3, B5, E, beta-carotene; calcium, copper, iron, magnesium, phosphate, zinc; fiber; ellagic acid, flavonoids

lemon & lime shot

A great wake-up call, this shot of citrus will give you a kickstart in the morning—the dash of lime gives it a real zing.

1 large lemon, halved
1 lime, halved

How to do it Squeeze the juice from the lemon and lime, stir together and serve immediately.

NUTRIENTS:
Packed with: vitamin C
Also contains: vitamin B complex

kiwi & apple

A classic apple juice with a twist that brings a subtle undercurrent of the lovely sweet kiwi flavor.

5 apples, stemmed and quartered
1 kiwi, peeled and halved

How to do it Put the apples through an electric juicer. Pour the juice into a blender or food processor, add the kiwi and blend until smooth. Serve immediately.

NUTRIENTS:
Packed with: vitamins B6, B7, C, beta-carotene; manganese
Plenty of: vitamins B2, B3; copper, phosphate, potassium, zinc; flavonoids
Also contains: calcium, magnesium, iron

The fresher the better

If you have the time to juice all your fruit and veg to make your juice cocktails, that's great. But you can use top-up juices too, from the refrigerated section.

kiwi & pine-lime

A great drink to freshen your skin and give it a healthy glow.

½ **pineapple, peeled and cut into chunks**
¼ **lime**
1 **kiwi, peeled and halved**

How to do it Put the pineapple through an electric juicer. (Alternatively, add ⅔ cup pineapple juice instead of juicing the pineapple.) Squeeze the juice from the lime. Pour the juices into a blender or food processor, add the kiwi and blend until smooth. Serve immediately.

NUTRIENTS:
Packed with: vitamin C; manganese
Plenty of: vitamins B1, B6; copper
Also contains:
vitamins B2, B3, B5, beta-carotene, folic acid; calcium, iron, magnesium, phosphate, potassium, zinc; fiber

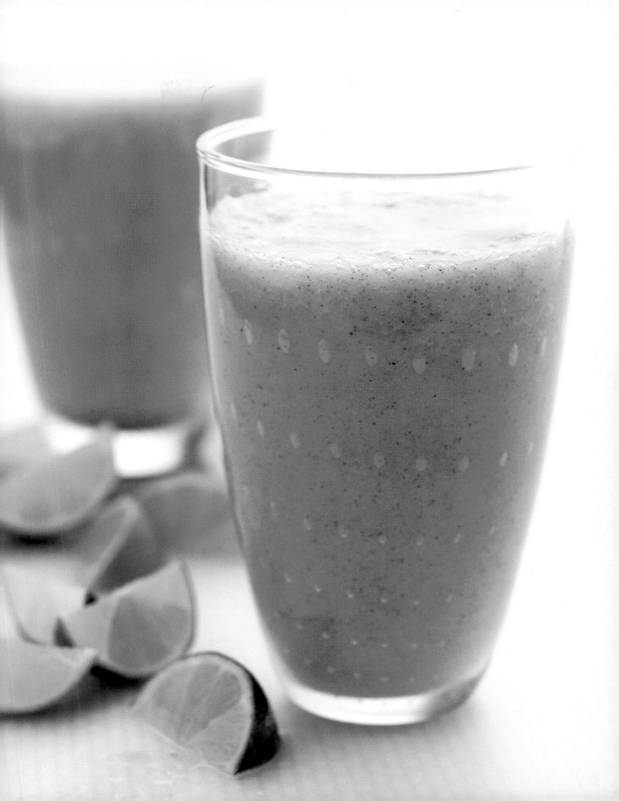

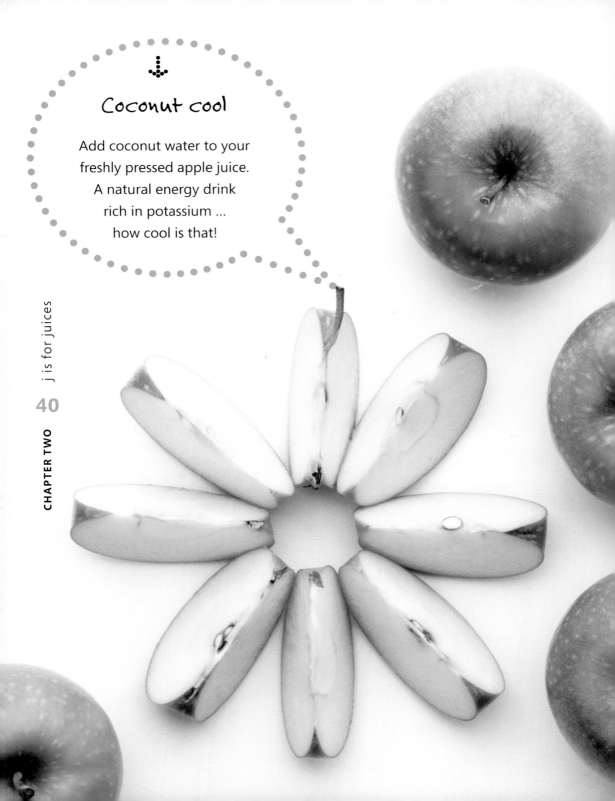

Coconut cool

Add coconut water to your
freshly pressed apple juice.
A natural energy drink
rich in potassium ...
how cool is that!

apple strawberry cooler

With its subtle pink color and delicate flavor, you could easily underestimate the power of this energy booster.

2 apples, stemmed and quartered
10 strawberries
⅔ cup coconut water

How to do it Put the apples through an electric juicer. Pour the juice into a blender or food processor, add the strawberries and coconut water and blend until smooth. Serve immediately.

NUTRIENTS:
Packed with: vitamin C; manganese
Also contains: vitamins B complex, E, beta-carotene, folic acid; calcium, copper, iron, magnesium, phosphate, potassium, zinc; fiber; ellagic acid, flavonoids

melon, mango & orange juice

A classic summer combination that's a good all-round burst of fruit goodness, whatever type of sweet melon you choose.

4 oranges, halved
2 pieces (about 1-inch cubes) peeled honeydew melon
½ mango, peeled and pitted

How to do it Squeeze the juice from the oranges. Pour the juice into a blender or food processor, add the melon and mango and blend until smooth and creamy. Serve immediately.

NUTRIENTS:
Packed with: vitamins B5, B6, C, beta-carotene; manganese, potassium
Plenty of: vitamins B1, B2, B3, B7, folic acid; copper, iron, magnesium, phosphate; fiber

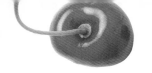

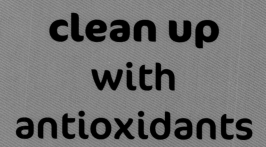

clean up with antioxidants

Do you want lustrous hair, glowing skin, and a mind that works double the speed of Mark Zuckerberg's? Don't we all! But the good news is that it is not as impossible as it may sound. The answer? Start juicing and fill up on antioxidants. These super-nutrients in fruit and vegetables protect your body from cell damage to your skin, your vital organs, and—most important of all—your brain. So get juicing, Maestro!

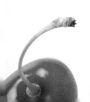

Why is that?

Chemical nasties called free radicals zip about your body damaging your cells, causing the signs of aging and compromising your optimum performance. Antioxidants seek them out, round them up and destroy them. So the more antioxidants you can pack into your diet, the healthier and more youthful you will be. The main antioxidant nutrients are:

- **Vitamin C**—provides the first line of defense.
- **Vitamin E**—this is the one that keeps you young.
- **Beta-carotene**—keeps you safe from the sun's rays.
- **Glutathione**—the ultimate warrior against toxins.
- **Flavonoids**—get the other antioxidants going.
- **Polyphenols**—keep those free radicals and other toxins in check.
- **Selenium**—fights against cell damage.

Free Radicals are not a new boy band

But antioxidants really do have the X factor.

It's a weird paradox that while we need oxygen for life, in metabolism it becomes a highly reactive molecule that damages our cells and our DNA.

If you want to mop up free radicals, don't just reach for an antioxidant supplement. Much, much better to juice a great rainbow selection of fruits and veggies. From red strawberries through green apples to the deepest purple plums, they'll give you something to sing about.

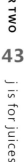

Hear me roar!

This juice really packs
a punch in the nutrition stakes.
Top up on your vitamin C
in one health-giving glass.
You'll be in great shape and
king of the concrete jungle.

citrus beast

Powerful by name and nature, this citrus
combo is a real fighter for great health.

3 oranges, halved
½ ruby grapefruit
½ lime
¼ lemon
8 cranberries

How to do it Squeeze the juice from
the oranges, grapefruit, lime and lemon.
(Alternatively, add ⅔ cup orange juice instead
of squeezing the oranges.) Pour the juices into a
blender or food processor, add the cranberries
and blend until smooth. Serve immediately.

NUTRIENTS:
Packed with: vitamin C
Plenty of: folic acid;
potassium
Also contains: vitamin
B complex, beta-
carotene; calcium, iron,
magnesium, manganese,
phosphate; flavonoids

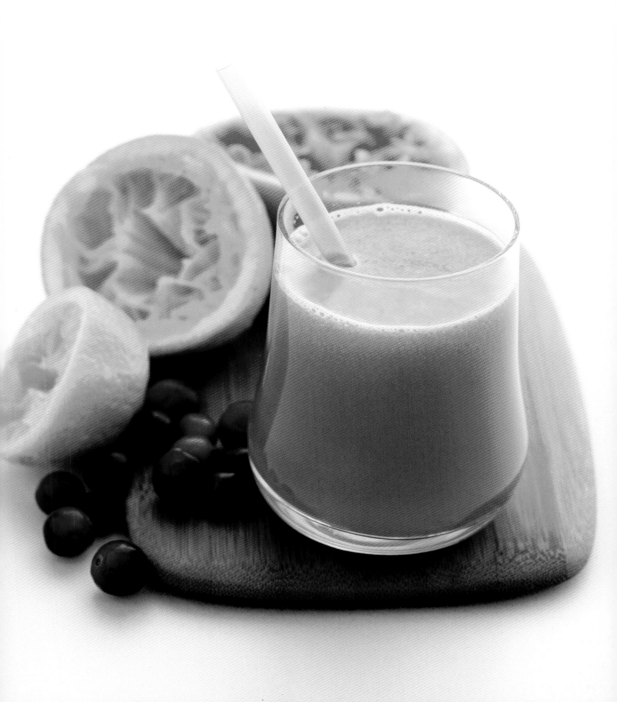

strawberry & mango

A naturally sweet duo juice with qualities that boost your brain function, ease stiff joints and protect your delicate eyesight.

½ cup strawberries
½ mango, peeled and pitted

✳ How to make a duo juice

NUTRIENTS:
Packed with: vitamins C, beta-carotene; copper, manganese; fiber
Plenty of: vitamins B5, B6, E; iron, magnesium, potassium
Also contains: vitamins B1, B2, B3, folic acid; calcium, phosphate, zinc; ellagic acid, flavonoids

✳ How to make a duo juice
Put all the fruit through an electric juicer. Stir in any top-up juices, if included, and serve immediately.

peach & raspberry

Banish fatigue and bring that youthful glow back to your skin with this rich and smooth duo juice.

6 peaches, pitted
1 handful of raspberries

✳ How to make a duo juice

NUTRIENTS:
Packed with: vitamins B2, B3, B5, C, beta-carotene; copper, iron, magnesium, manganese, phosphate, potassium; fiber
Plenty of: vitamins B1, folic acid; iodine
Also contains: vitamins E, B7; calcium, zinc; ellagic acid, flavonoids

lychee coco

Deliciously oriental, try this exotic duo combination to give your circulation a vital boost.

10 canned lychees
⅔ cup coconut water

✱ How to make a duo juice

   NUTRIENTS:
   Packed with: vitamin C; copper
   Plenty of: calcium
   Also contains: vitamins B2, B6, folic acid; iron, magnesium, manganese, phosphate, potassium, zinc; fiber

squelch juice

With its powerful antioxidants, this punchy duo juice can help tone up your digestive system. If you prefer, you can blend the grapes, then enjoy the satisfying squelch as you pass the juice through a strainer.

9 ounces seedless red grapes
9 ounces seedless green grapes

✱ How to make a duo juice

   NUTRIENTS:
   Packed with: vitamins B1, B6, C; copper, manganese, potassium
   Plenty of: beta-carotene; iron, magnesium, phosphate; fiber
   Also contains: vitamins B2, B3, B5, B7, folic acid; calcium, zinc; flavonoids, iodine

"You ol' limey!"

Gone are the days when they used to carry limes on board ship to prevent the sailors suffering from scurvy. But you still shouldn't neglect your vitamin C, so here's a healthy shot just in case ...

lucky limes

For a bright smile and a healthy digestive system, try your luck with this great mix of soft and sharp flavors.

½ pineapple, peeled and cut into chunks
3 limes, halved
½ mango, peeled and pitted

How to do it Put the pineapple through an electric juicer. Squeeze the juice from the limes. Pour the juices into a blender or food processor, add the mango and blend until smooth and creamy. Serve immediately.

NUTRIENTS:
Packed with: vitamins B6, C, beta-carotene; copper, manganese
Plenty of: vitamins B1, B2, B3, B5; magnesium, potassium; fiber
Also contains: vitamins B7, E, folic acid; calcium, iron, phosphate, zinc; flavonoids

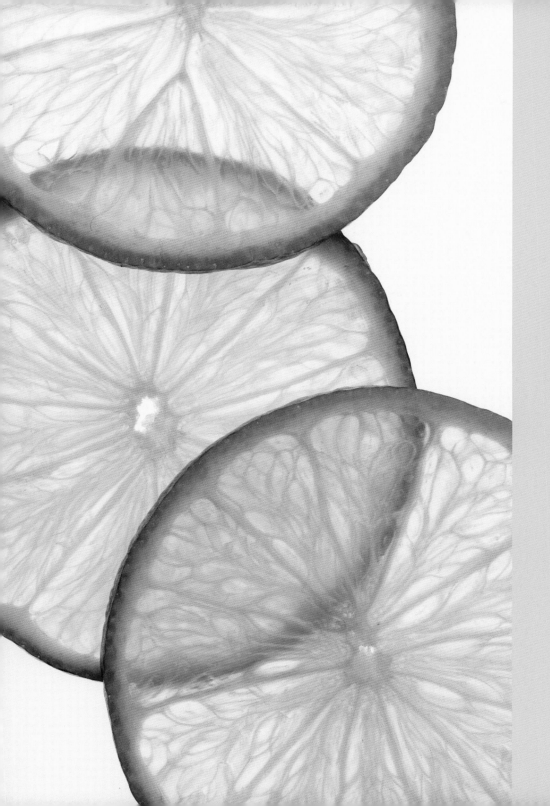

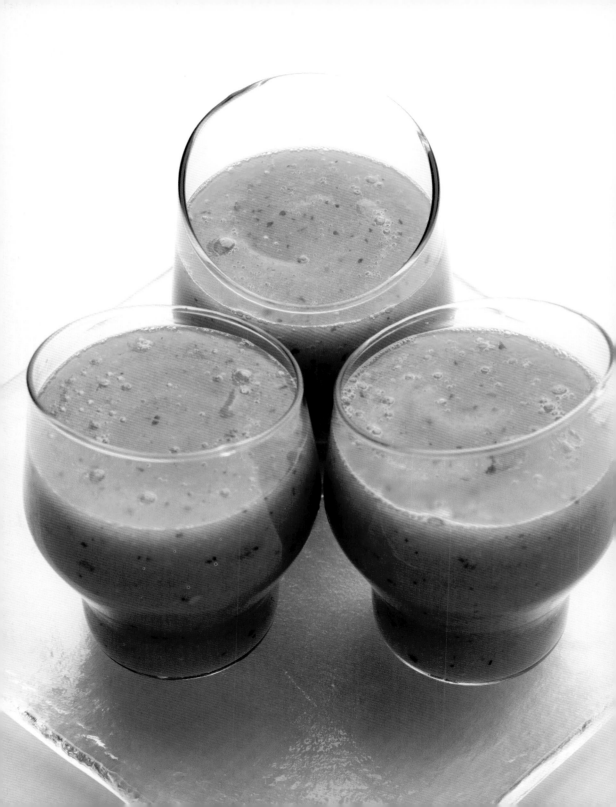

"Wasabi, doc?"

With mint and pineapple,
this is a marriage made in heaven.
You don't juice the papaya seeds but
there's no need to waste them.
They are edible and
have a peppery taste
like wasabi.

bali baby

Be my Bali baby with this mint-fresh juice—a real digestive soother.

½ pineapple, peeled and cut into chunks
¼ papaya, peeled and seeded
3 mint leaves

How to do it Put the pineapple through an electric juicer. Pour the juice into a blender or food processor, add the papaya and mint leaves and blend until smooth and the leaves are finely chopped. (Alternatively, you can simply chop the mint leaves and add them to the juice.)
Serve immediately.

NUTRIENTS:
Packed with: vitamins B1, C, beta-carotene; copper, magnesium, manganese
Plenty of: vitamins B2, B5, B6; iron, phosphate, potassium, zinc
Also contains: vitamins B3, B7, E, folic acid; calcium; fiber; flavonoids

orange ginger jazz

Soothe your muscles and restore your system with this jazzy combination.

3 thin slices ginger root
1½ pears, stemmed and quartered
3 oranges, halved

How to do it Put the ginger and pears through an electric juicer. Squeeze the juice from the oranges. Stir the juices together and serve immediately.

NUTRIENTS:
Packed with: vitamins B1, C, folic acid; copper, magnesium, potassium
Plenty of: vitamins B2, B3, B5, B6, E; iron, phosphate
Also contains: beta-carotene; calcium, zinc

vital start

Sharpen your senses, refresh your system and absorb slow-release energy to see you through a busy day at work.

1 piece (about 1-inch cube) peeled pineapple
3 oranges, halved
1 banana
1½ kiwis, peeled and halved

How to do it Put the pineapple through an electric juicer. Squeeze the juice from the oranges. Pour the juices into a blender or food processor, add the remaining ingredients and blend until smooth and creamy. Serve immediately.

NUTRIENTS:
Packed with: vitamins A, B1, B2, B6, C, K, folic acid; copper, magnesium, manganese, potassium
Plenty of: vitamin B5; calcium, iron, phosphate
Also contains: vitamin E; fiber

pear & ginger

With their smooth and subtle flavor, pears quietly get to work protecting you from toxins and cell damage.

5 pears, stemmed and quartered
2 thin slices ginger root

How to do it Put all the ingredients through an electric juicer. Stir the juices together and serve immediately.

NUTRIENTS:
Packed with: copper, magnesium, potassium
Plenty of: vitamins B2, B3, B5, B6, C, E; iron, phosphate
Also contains: vitamins B1, beta-carotene, folic acid; calcium, zinc

cloudy apple & mint

Flush impurities out of your system by marrying your freshly juiced apples with the wonderful lift of fresh mint.

6 apples, stemmed and quartered
5 mint leaves

How to do it Put the apples through an electric juicer. Pour the juice into a blender or food processor, add the mint leaves and blend until smooth and the leaves are finely chopped. (Alternatively, you can simply chop the mint leaves and add them to the juice.) Serve immediately.

NUTRIENTS:
Packed with: manganese
Plenty of: vitamins B1, B6, B7, C, beta-carotene; potassium
Also contains: vitamins B2, B3, E; calcium, copper, iron, magnesium, phosphate, zinc; flavonoids

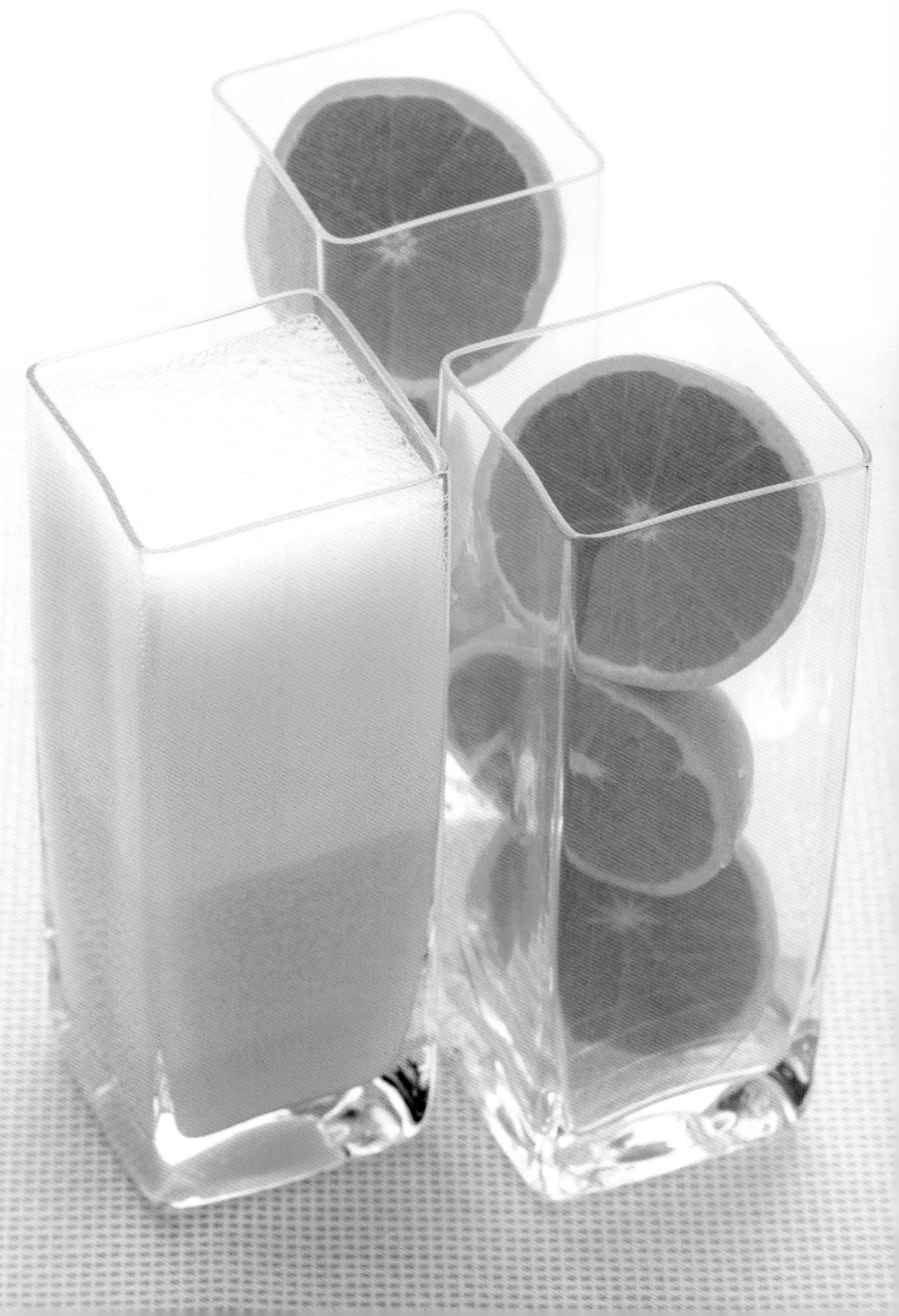

So that's what it is!

How many times have you walked past that
pale-green basketball-sized fruit
and wondered what it is?
Now you know!
Try using the pomelo peel
to make marmalade.
It's fabulous!

pomelo tango

With a sweeter, milder flavor than its
cousin the grapefruit, the pomelo gives
citrus juice a whole new dimension. But you
can use grapefruit instead if you cannot
find a pomelo.

1 pomelo, halved
1 tangerine, halved
½ lime

How to do it Squeeze the juice from
the fruits. Stir the juices together and serve
immediately.

NUTRIENTS:
Packed with: vitamin C
Also contains:
vitamins B complex,
beta-carotene, folic
acid; calcium, iron,
magnesium, manganese,
phosphate, potassium;
flavonoids

hot apple & cinnamon

This lovely warming spice can help fight those winter colds and keep up your resistance to infection.

5 apples, stemmed and quartered
1 teaspoon ground cinnamon

How to do it Put the apples through an electric juicer and stir in the cinnamon. Warm the juice in a pan over low heat and serve immediately.

NUTRIENTS:
Packed with: vitamins B1, B6, B7, C, beta-carotene; potassium
Plenty of: vitamins B2, B3, E; copper, iron, magnesium, phosphate, zinc

raspberry coco

Smooth the way through your system and boost your energy levels with a hit of pink power.

½ cup raspberries
1 cup coconut water
3 mint leaves

How to do it Put all the ingredients in a blender or food processor and blend until smooth and the mint leaves are finely chopped. (Alternatively, you can simply chop the mint leaves and add them to the juice.) Serve immediately.

NUTRIENTS:
Packed with: vitamin C, manganese
Also contains: vitamins B1, B2, B3, B5, B6, B7, E, folic acid; calcium, copper, iron, magnesium, phosphate, potassium, zinc; fiber; ellagic acid, flavonoids

pear & ginger cleanser

Cleanse your body of harmful free radicals and soothe your system with this crisp and clean mix.

3 pears, stemmed and quartered
2 thin slices ginger root
¼ cucumber

How to do it Put all the ingredients through an electric juicer. Stir the juices together and serve immediately.

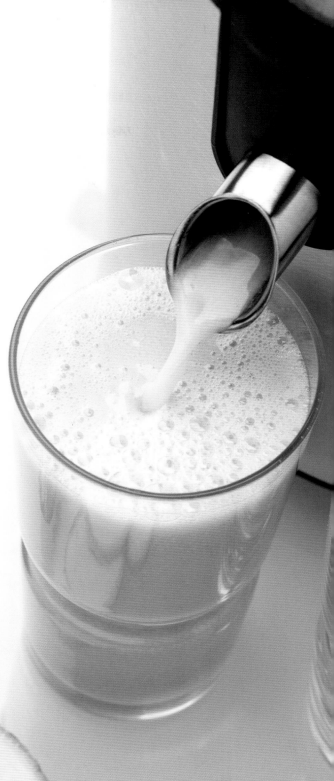

NUTRIENTS:
Packed with: vitamins B5, B6, C, beta-carotene; copper, magnesium, phosphate, potassium
Plenty of: vitamins B1, B2, B3, B7, E, folic acid; calcium, iron, zinc
Also contains: vitamin K; flavonoids; omega-3

It's not for your face ... before you ask

bounce with energy

Juice is pure, unfiltered energy. It's a divinely and deliciously guilt-free high—no caffeine, no chemicals, no nasty refined sugar—just raw, unadulterated, healthy and flavor-filled bounce. Every day your energy levels go up and down. A coffee or a candy bar are ultimately unsatisfactory quick fixes for those inevitable troughs, but if you drink down a fresh juice, you'll burst with zing and hold the high for hours. No nasties, just goodness and loads of sustainable energy.

Charge me up, baby!

Okay, be honest—how long do you feel buzzed after a sneaky bar of chocolate? Was it really worth it? The good news is that if you choose the right juice blend you'll keep going a heck of a lot longer than your smartphone (which isn't saying much, it's true).

For your **potassium** needs, a banana always does the trick, as well as providing natural sweetness. It keeps your muscles moving and turns them into tanks for carbohydrates, your body's primary fuel.

You'll need **iron**, too, to transport oxygen to your cells; you can't keep powering forward without it.

And then there's **selenium**—it packs power into every cell, giving you a spring in your step.

Where do we get all that?

When you want to juice for bounce, choose juices that include the high-energy boosters, and mix the colors of the fruit and veg you choose for the maximum impact.

You'll get a pure-power blast from the hot spectrum colors: red is for go in the nutrients context.

GO RED—to give your body a bounce by juicing apples, cherries, grapes, redcurrants, strawberries, tomatoes.

> **GO AMBER**—to maintain that energy high by juicing apricots, bananas, lemons, mangoes, papayas, peaches.

Choose your seasons

Juice fruit and veggies at their best.
When plums are ripe and in season,
they are at their juiciest—and
bursting with the
vitamins and minerals
we are looking for.

ginger plum

If you are hoping to preserve your
youthful looks and energy, there is
nothing better than trying a ginger
plum juice now and then.

2 thin slices ginger root
5 oranges, halved
2 plums, peeled and pitted

How to do it Put the ginger through
an electric juicer. Squeeze the juice from the
oranges. Pour the juices into a blender or
food processor, add the plums and blend until
smooth. Serve immediately.

NUTRIENTS:
Packed with: vitamin C,
beta-carotene; copper,
manganese, potassium
Plenty of: vitamins B3,
B5, B6; magnesium,
phosphate
Also contains: vitamins
B1, B2, B7, E, K, folic acid;
calcium, iron, zinc; fiber;
flavonoids, omega-3

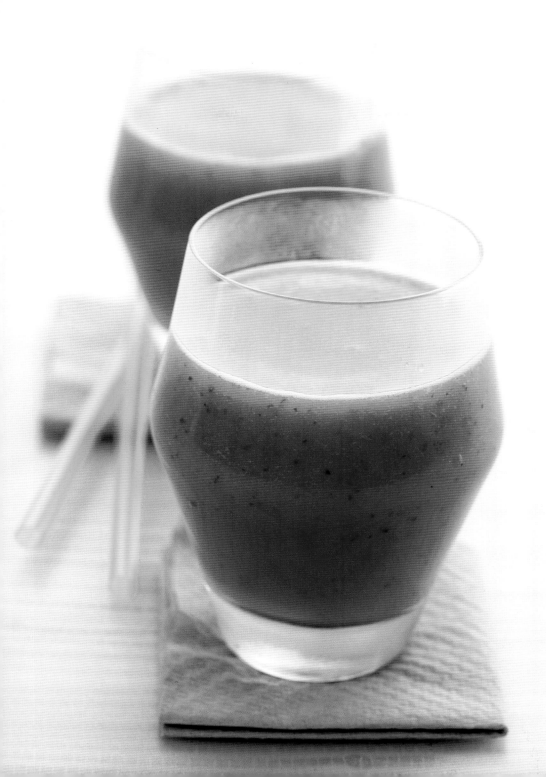

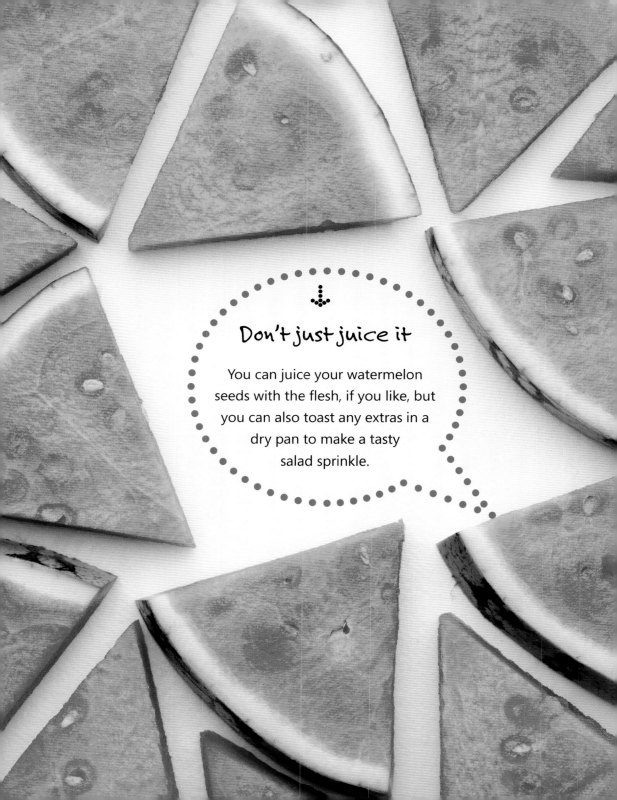

Don't just juice it

You can juice your watermelon
seeds with the flesh, if you like, but
you can also toast any extras in a
dry pan to make a tasty
salad sprinkle.

watermelon refresher

Refreshing and stimulating, this is a real brightening juice that is ideal for breakfast or lunch.

½ watermelon, peeled, seeded and cut into chunks
¼ cucumber
6 strawberries
3 mint leaves

How to do it Put the watermelon and cucumber through an electric juicer. Pour the juices into a blender or food processor, add the strawberries and mint leaves and blend until smooth and the leaves are finely chopped. (Alternatively, you can simply chop the mint leaves and add them to the juice.) Serve immediately.

NUTRIENTS:
Packed with: vitamins B5, B6, C, beta-carotene
Plenty of: vitamins B1, B3, B7; magnesium, phosphate, potassium, zinc
Also contains: vitamins B2, E, folic acid; calcium, copper, iron, manganese; fiber; ellagic acid, flavonoids

grapefruit kickstarter

No surprises here—the perfect breakfast juice combo if you need a boost to get your day started. Add half a chili if you dare!

2 large grapefruits, halved
½ lime
3 mint leaves
¼ chili

How to do it Squeeze the juice from the grapefruits and lime. Pour the juices into a blender or food processor, add the mint leaves and chili and blend until smooth and the leaves are finely chopped. (Alternatively, you can simply chop the mint leaves and add them to the juice.) Serve immediately.

NUTRIENTS:
Packed with: vitamins C, folic acid
Plenty of: vitamins B1, B7; calcium, magnesium, phosphate, potassium
Also contains: vitamins B2, B3, B5, B6, E, beta-carotene; copper, iron; flavonoids

tropfest

Imagine yourself on a tropical island while you indulge in this exotic concoction.

2 pieces (about 2-inch cubes) peeled pineapple
½ watermelon, peeled, seeded and cut into chunks
1 slice (1 inch thick) papaya, peeled and seeded
3 mint leaves

How to do it Put all the fruit through an electric juicer. Pour the juices into a blender or food processor, add the mint leaves and blend until smooth and the leaves are finely chopped. (Alternatively, you can simply chop the mint leaves and add them to the juice.) Serve immediately.

> **NUTRIENTS:**
> **Packed with:** vitamins B1, B5, B7, C, beta-carotene; magnesium, manganese, phosphate, potassium
> **Plenty of:** vitamin B2; calcium, copper, zinc
> **Also contains:** vitamins B3, E, folic acid; fiber; flavonoids

pineapple, thai basil & lime

Great for your digestion, this fresh-tasting juice will also brighten your complexion and flush out your system.

½ pineapple, peeled and cut into chunks
¼ lime
1 small handful of Thai basil leaves

How to do it Put the pineapple through an electric juicer. Squeeze the juice from the lime. Pour the juices into a blender or food processor, add the basil leaves and blend until smooth and the leaves are finely chopped. (Alternatively, you can simply chop the basil leaves and add them to the juice.) Serve immediately.

> **NUTRIENTS:**
> **Packed with:** vitamin C; manganese
> **Plenty of:** vitamins B1, B6
> **Also contains:** vitamins B3, B5, folic acid; calcium, copper, iron, magnesium, potassium, zinc

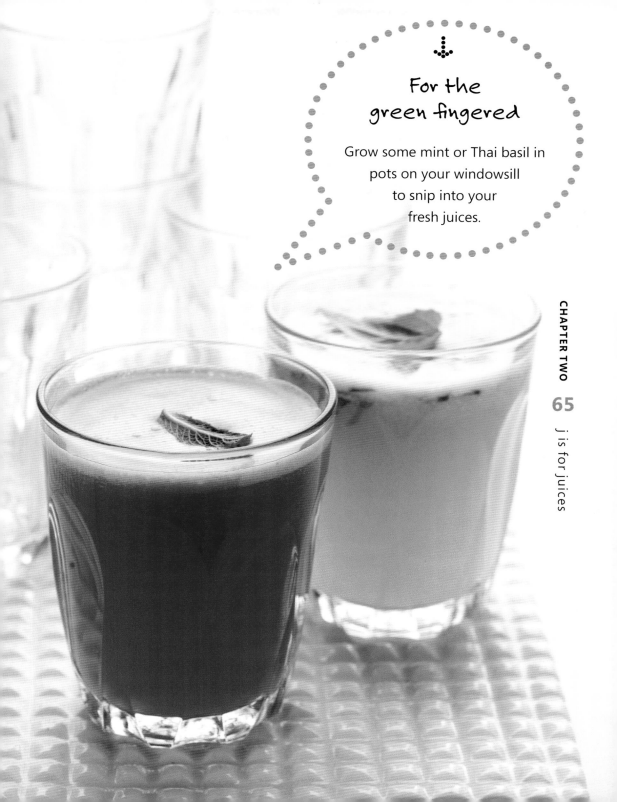

For the green fingered

Grow some mint or Thai basil in pots on your windowsill to snip into your fresh juices.

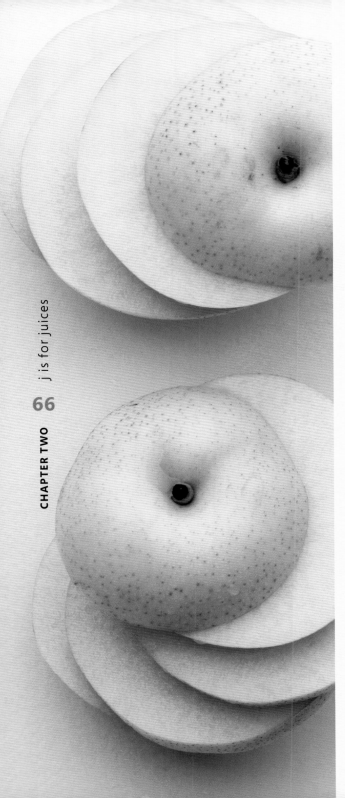

yuzu & asian pear

Japanese pears have a subtle flavor and digestive-cleansing qualities. If you can't find yuzu juice, you can use lime juice instead.

**6 Asian pears, quartered
    and stems removed
2 teaspoons yuzu or lime juice**

How to do it Put the Asian pears through an electric juicer. Stir the yuzu into the juice and serve immediately.

NUTRIENTS:
Packed with: vitamins C, folic acid; manganese, potassium
Plenty of: copper, magnesium
Also contains: vitamin K

pink grapefruit & ginger

The humble grapefruit is a great way to stimulate your body first thing in the morning, boosting the immune system and getting you ready for the day.

2 thin slices ginger root
3 pink grapefruits, halved

How to do it Put the ginger through an electric juicer. Squeeze the juice from the grapefruits. Stir the juices together and serve immediately.

NUTRIENTS:
Packed with: vitamins B1, B5, B6, C; copper, magnesium, phosphate, potassium
Plenty of: vitamins B3, beta-carotene; calcium
Also contains: vitamin B2; iron, zinc; flavonoids; limonene

watermelon & mint

Freshen your breath and clear your head with this delicious combination.

½ watermelon, peeled, seeded and cut into chunks
5 mint leaves

How to do it Put the watermelon through an electric juicer. Pour the juice into a blender or food processor, add the mint leaves and blend until smooth and the leaves are finely chopped. (Alternatively, you can simply chop the mint leaves and add them to the juice.) Serve immediately.

NUTRIENTS:
Packed with: vitamins B1, B5, B6, C, beta-carotene
Plenty of: vitamin B7; copper, iron, magnesium, potassium, zinc
Also contains: vitamins B2, B3; calcium, phosphate

zesty citrus fruits

Better than a Norwegian ice bath to wake you up first thing in the morning, citrus juice works wonders after a late night. And when everyone else is sinking cocktails but you want to be virtuous, try adding sparkling mineral water to citrus juice for a healthy spritzer. And the really good news? You won't get that office cold that's been going around.

Tell me more ...

Did you know that an orange contains a full dose of your Recommended Dietary Allowance of vitamin C? One orange. Amazing. Quite simply, citrus fruits look after you in ways that no other foods can. They are packed not only with high levels of vitamin C, but also folate, phytonutrients and potassium. Who needs a doctor?

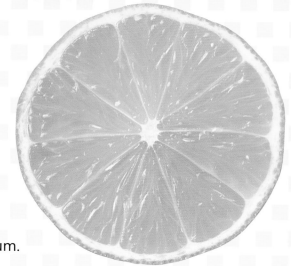

What will all that do for me?

- **Boost immunity**—keep those coughs and colds at arm's length. Studies show that the high levels of vitamin C may even protect against long-term health problems.

- **Heal wounds**—vitamin C helps speed up collagen formation, the stuff that binds together our skin.

- **Nurture cells**—the folate (a B vitamin) in citrus fruits is known to promote new cell growth and the formation of DNA (your genetic code). If you're pregnant, make sure you get enough to help protect your developing baby.

- **Heal your heart**—the nutrients in citrus fruits have been shown to lower blood pressure, helping keep the negative effects of stress at bay.

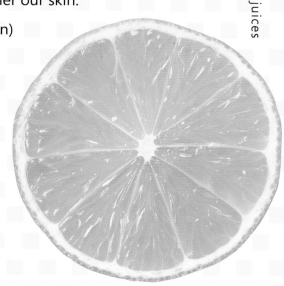

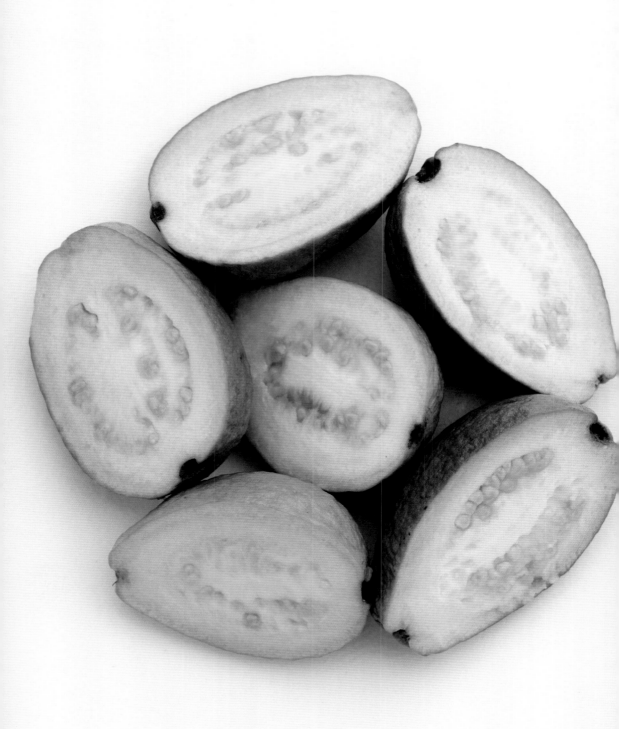

guava thai

Distinctly Asian in style, this sharply delicious mix will transport you to tropical Thai heaven. Use two handfuls of strawberries if you cannot find a guava, and just put the lime juice and all the ingredients in a blender.

½ guava, peeled
½ lime
1 cup coconut water
1 kaffir lime leaf

How to do it Put the guava through an electric juicer. Squeeze the juice from the lime. Pour the juices into a blender or food processor, add the coconut water and the kaffir lime leaf and blend until smooth and the leaf is finely chopped. (Alternatively, you can simply chop the lime leaf and add it to the juice.) Serve immediately.

NUTRIENTS:
Packed with: vitamins C, beta-carotene
Plenty of: potassium
Also contains: vitamin B complex; calcium, copper, iron, magnesium, phosphate

fall cleanser

Purify your blood and refresh your spirit with this fall fruit combination.

3 apples, stemmed and quartered
3 pears, stemmed and quartered
2 thin slices ginger root

How to do it Put all the ingredients through an electric juicer. Stir the juices together and serve immediately.

NUTRIENTS:
Packed with: vitamins B6, C; copper, magnesium, manganese, potassium
Plenty of: vitamins B1, B2, B3, B7, E, beta-carotene; phosphate, zinc; fiber
Also contains: vitamins B5, K, folic acid; calcium; flavonoids, omega-3

Something to tell your teacher

A real superfood, did you know that guavas have four times more antioxidants than apples?

Small but mighty

Don't let yourself be fooled by modest appearances. Tiny tamarillos contain lycopene—a flavonoid that's a powerful ally in the fight against free radicals.

tamarillo apple

The tamarillo is known as the "tree tomato." Halve the fruit and scoop out the flesh to capture its health-giving properties. You can use two tomatoes instead if a tamarillo is hard to find.

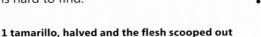

1 tamarillo, halved and the flesh scooped out
3 apples, stemmed and quartered
¼ pineapple, peeled and cut into chunks
3 mint leaves

How to do it Put the tamarillo, apples and pineapple through an electric juicer. Pour the juices into a blender or food processor, add the mint leaves and blend until smooth and the leaves are finely chopped. (Alternatively, you can simply chop the mint leaves and add them to the juice.) Serve immediately.

NUTRIENTS:
Packed with: vitamin C
Plenty of: vitamins B1, B6, B7, beta-carotene; copper, manganese, potassium
Also contains: vitamins B2, B3, B5, E, folic acid; calcium, iron, magnesium, phosphate, zinc; flavonoids

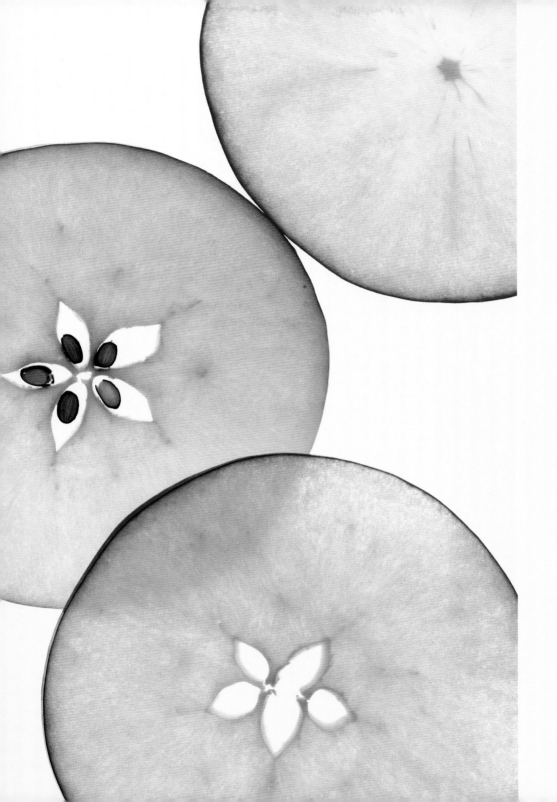

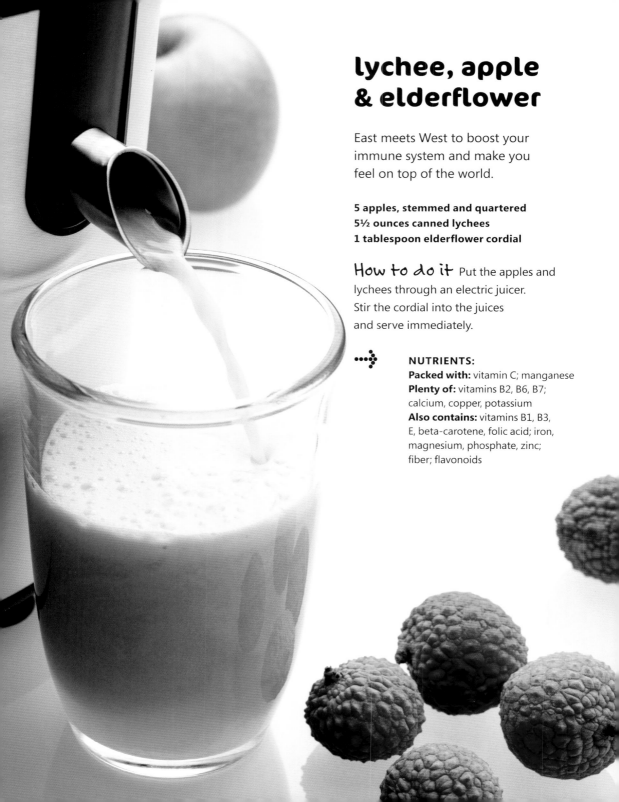

lychee, apple & elderflower

East meets West to boost your immune system and make you feel on top of the world.

5 apples, stemmed and quartered
5½ ounces canned lychees
1 tablespoon elderflower cordial

How to do it Put the apples and lychees through an electric juicer. Stir the cordial into the juices and serve immediately.

NUTRIENTS:
Packed with: vitamin C; manganese
Plenty of: vitamins B2, B6, B7; calcium, copper, potassium
Also contains: vitamins B1, B3, E, beta-carotene, folic acid; iron, magnesium, phosphate, zinc; fiber; flavonoids

Kale is king—and the Champion juicer's favorite veggie

sunday glory

Start your Sunday morning with a leisurely read of the newspapers and a glass of this combo to take you through the day stress-free and revitalized.

3 pieces (about 1-inch cubes) peeled pineapple
2 apples, stemmed and quartered
3 oranges, halved
12 strawberries

How to do it Put the pineapple and apples through an electric juicer. Squeeze the juice from the oranges. Pour the juices into a blender or food processor, add the strawberries and blend until smooth. Serve immediately.

NUTRIENTS:
Packed with: vitamins B1, B6, C, folic acid; magnesium, manganese, potassium
Plenty of: vitamins A, B2, B5; calcium, copper, iron, phosphate
Also contains: omega-3, selenium

core-d cleanse

Kale really packs a nutritional punch, so keep it in your juicing repertoire and love its anti-aging properties.

½ pineapple, peeled and cut into chunks
1 handful of kale
¼ cucumber
¼ lemon
½ avocado, peeled and pitted

How to do it Put the pineapple, kale and cucumber through an electric juicer. (Alternatively, add ⅔ cup pineapple juice instead of juicing the pineapple.) Squeeze the juice from the lemon. Pour the juices into a blender or food processor, add the avocado and blend until smooth and creamy. Serve immediately.

NUTRIENTS:
Packed with: vitamins B1, B2, B5, B6, B7, C, E, beta-carotene; magnesium, manganese, phosphate, potassium
Plenty of: vitamins B3, folic acid; calcium, copper, iron, zinc
Also contains: vitamin K; fiber; iodine

Natural highs

Juicing gives an instant energy hit
without the usual suspects
of refined sugars
and caffeine.

lean green

Lean Green is probably the tastiest juice
you'll come across that's made with kale.
Kale is packed so full of nutrients that we've
always wanted to find a way to make it taste
good in a juice. For us, the combination
of the kiwi and pineapple balance out the
metallic nature of the kale and spinach.
A fantastic juice to get you going first
thing in the morning.

2 green apples, stemmed and quartered
1 handful of baby spinach leaves
1 handful of kale
1 pear, stemmed and quartered
2 pieces (about 1-inch cubes) peeled pineapple
1 kiwi, peeled and halved

How to do it Put all the ingredients
through an electric juicer. Stir the juices together
and serve immediately.

NUTRIENTS:
Packed with: vitamins
B1, B2, B6, C, beta-
carotene; copper,
magnesium, manganese,
potassium
Plenty of: vitamins
B3, B5, B7, folic acid;
calcium, iron
Also contains: vitamins
E, K; zinc; flavonoids;
iodine

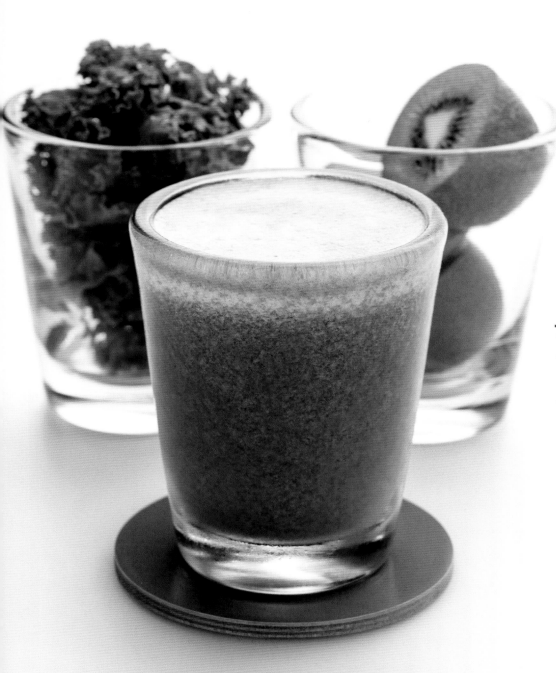

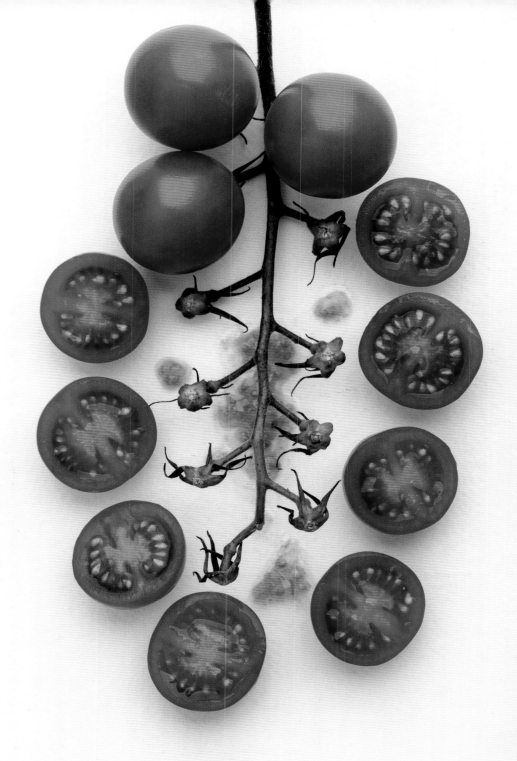

veggie invigorator

Packed with antioxidants to flush those free radicals out of your system, the delicious carrot juice is boosted with a touch of spicy ginger.

3 carrots, tops removed
2 tomatoes
½ rib celery
2 thin slices ginger root
½ lemon

How to do it Put all the ingredients except the lemon through an electric juicer. Squeeze the juice from the lemon. Stir the juices together and serve immediately.

> **NUTRIENTS:**
> **Packed with:** vitamins B1, B6, B7, C, E, beta-carotene; magnesium, manganese, phosphate, potassium
> **Plenty of:** vitamins B3; calcium, iron
> **Also contains:** vitamin B2; zinc; iodine

mango & carrot

This could surely be the sunniest juice on offer and it's guaranteed to brighten your day.

10 carrots, tops removed
½ mango, peeled and pitted

How to do it Put the carrots through an electric juicer. Pour the juice into a blender or food processor, add the mango and blend until smooth and creamy. Serve immediately.

> **NUTRIENTS:**
> **Packed with:** vitamins B1, B5, B6, B7, C, E, beta-carotene, folic acid; calcium, copper, iron, manganese, phosphate, potassium
> **Plenty of:** vitamins B2, B3; magnesium, zinc; iodine

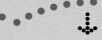

Red hot juice

Juices made with carrots are red hot in nutrients. Soften with mango for a creamy blend. Hit with tomatoes and they really rock.

classic orange & beet

Cut through with the tang of citrus, this anytime juice gives you natural energy combined with great blood purifying qualities.

1 beet
6 oranges, halved
1 lemon, halved

How to do it Put the beet through an electric juicer. Squeeze the juice from the oranges and lemon. Stir the juices together and serve immediately.

NUTRIENTS:
Packed with: vitamins B6, B7, C, beta-carotene, folic acid; magnesium, manganese, phosphate
Plenty of: vitamins B1, B2, B5; iron, potassium
Also contains: vitamin B3; zinc; limonene

super greens

With this combination, you are getting a complete health hit in a glass, bursting with vitamins, minerals and antioxidants to boost your system to perform to the max.

2 green apples, stemmed and quartered
1 handful of baby spinach leaves
1 handful of kale
1 kiwi, peeled and halved
1 pear, stemmed and quartered
1 piece (about 2 inches) cucumber
¼ lime

How to do it Put all the ingredients except the lime through an electric juicer. Squeeze the juice from the lime. Stir the juices together and serve immediately.

NUTRIENTS:
Packed with: vitamin C, beta-carotene; magnesium, phosphate, potassium
Plenty of: vitamins B1, B2, B5, B6, folic acid; calcium, iron
Also contains: vitamins B3, B7, E, K; zinc; flavonoids; iodine

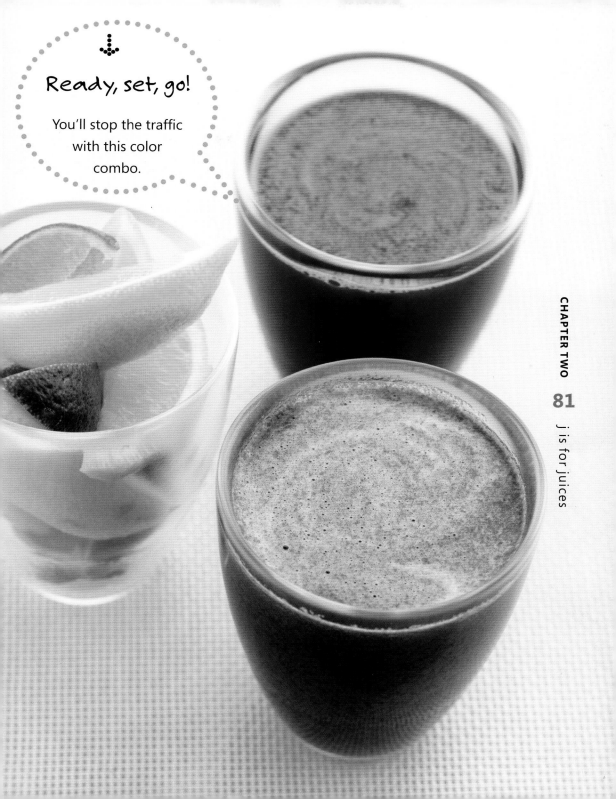

Ready, set, go!

You'll stop the traffic with this color combo.

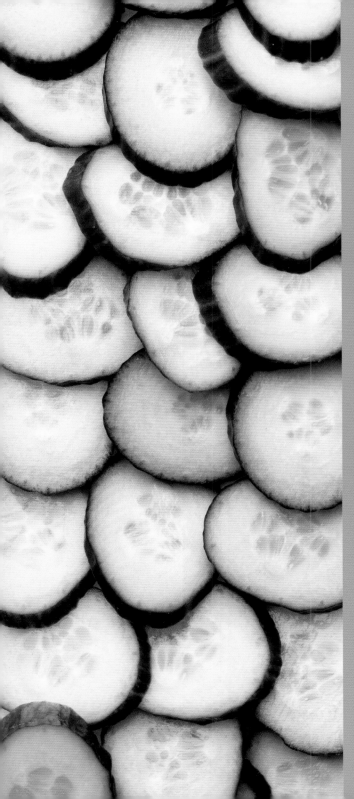

honeydew & cucumber

A glorious combination to boost your muscles and protect your heart.

½ honeydew melon, peeled and cut into chunks
¼ cucumber

How to do it Put all the ingredients through an electric juicer. Stir the juices together and serve immediately.

NUTRIENTS:
Packed with: vitamins B1, B5, B6, C, beta-carotene; magnesium, phosphate, potassium
Plenty of: calcium, iron; fiber
Also contains: vitamins B2, B7, E, folic acid; iodine

energizer

An imaginative juice boost, this will lift your energy levels, relax your muscles and put the spring back in your step.

3 apples, stemmed and quartered
3 carrots, tops removed
2 thin slices ginger root

How to do it
Put all the ingredients through an electric juicer. Stir the juices together and serve immediately.

NUTRIENTS:
Packed with: vitamins B1, B6, C, beta-carotene; copper, magnesium, manganese, phosphate, potassium
Plenty of: vitamins B3, B5, B7, E; calcium, iron, zinc
Also contains: vitamins B2, K, folic acid; iodine, selenium; flavonoids; omega-3

orange & carrot

Packed with beta-carotene and vitamin C, here's a juice to boost your immune system.

5 carrots, tops removed
3 oranges, halved

How to do it
Put the carrots through an electric juicer. Squeeze the juice from the oranges. Stir the juices together and serve immediately.

NUTRIENTS:
Packed with: vitamins B1, B5, B6, C, E, beta-carotene, folic acid; manganese, potassium
Plenty of: vitamin B7; iron, phosphate

raw juice

Eat plenty of raw foods to increase your nutrient intake to the max—or just juice 'em.

5 apples, stemmed and quartered
½ rib celery
½ lime
3 mint leaves

How to do it Put the apples and celery through an electric juicer. Squeeze the juice from the lime. Pour the juices into a blender or food processor, add the mint leaves and blend until smooth and the leaves are finely chopped. (Alternatively, you can simply chop the mint leaves and add them to the juice.) Serve immediately.

NUTRIENTS:
Packed with: vitamin C; manganese
Plenty of: vitamins B7, beta-carotene
Also contains: vitamins B1, B2, B3, E, folic acid; calcium, copper, iron, magnesium, phosphate, potassium, zinc; fiber; flavonoids

ginger zinger

You'll be zinging with antioxidants from this great combination—the squeeze of lime juice gives everything that final zing.

3 thin slices ginger root
4 carrots, tops removed
3 oranges, halved
½ lime

How to do it Put the ginger and carrots through an electric juicer. Squeeze the juice from the oranges and lime. Stir the juices together and serve immediately.

NUTRIENTS:
Packed with: vitamins A, B1, C, folic acid; magnesium, potassium
Plenty of: vitamins B2, B5, B6; calcium, iron
Also contains: phosphate

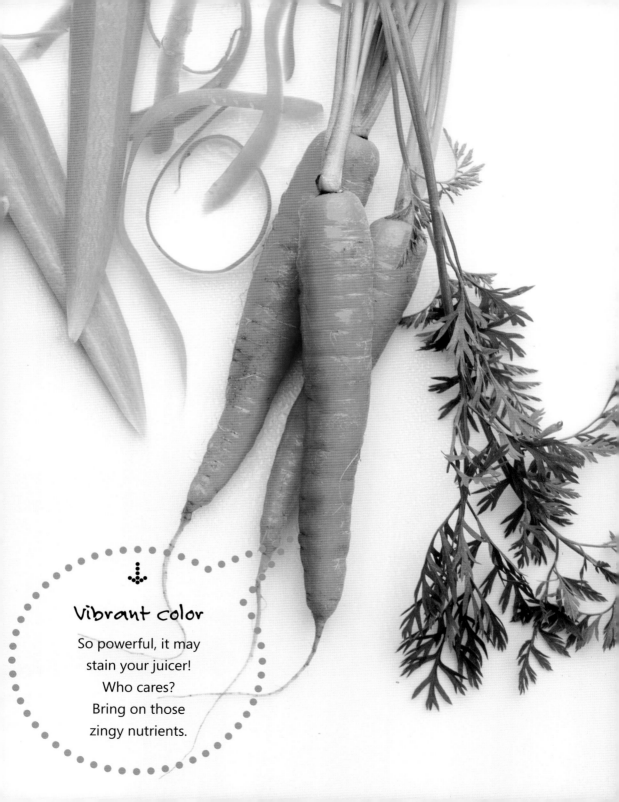

Vibrant color

So powerful, it may
stain your juicer!
Who cares?
Bring on those
zingy nutrients.

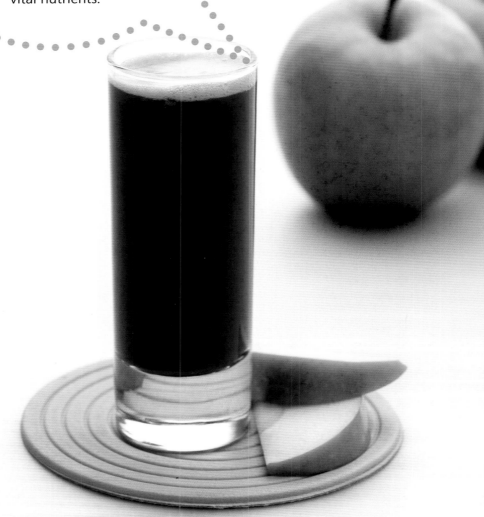

For best results, drink every day

Just 1 ounce of wheatgrass is the nutritional equivalent of eating 3 pounds of vegetables! The nutrients in wheatgrass get rid of toxins and replace them with vital nutrients.

wheatgrass shot

Used by ancient cultures 2,000 years ago for its regenerative and spiritual properties, wheatgrass grows from red wheatberry sprouts. One of nature's richest sources of nutrients, wheatgrass is packed with chlorophyll, active enzymes and vitamins A, C, E, B12 and B17.

1 tray wheatgrass
½ apple, cored and cut into wedges

How to do it Put the wheatgrass through a masticating juicer and pour into a glass. Serve immediately with the apple wedges. Take a sip of juice, then a bite of apple. You'll find the flavors and textures complement each other perfectly.

NUTRIENTS:
Packed with: vitamins A, C; iron
Plenty of: vitamins E, B12, B17; calcium, potassium

Here are 10 exciting reasons to make wheatgrass part of your daily routine

- It will boost your energy and help banish fatigue.
- Your body's metabolism will speed up and your appetite will reduce.
- Improved digestion means you'll get all the goodness from the food you eat.
- Wheatgrass juice helps lower blood pressure, enrich the blood and banish blood disorders.
- An antibacterial, it also flushes toxins out of the liver.
- Smile—wheatgrass can help prevent tooth decay.
- It's good for skin problems, improves your complexion and reduces acne.
- It eliminates dandruff and helps your hair to retain its natural color.
- Boosting the immune system and calming the nervous system are both sound benefits.
- The chlorophyll present in wheatgrass will neutralize and cleanse toxins from your body, help purify your liver, and fight the signs of aging.

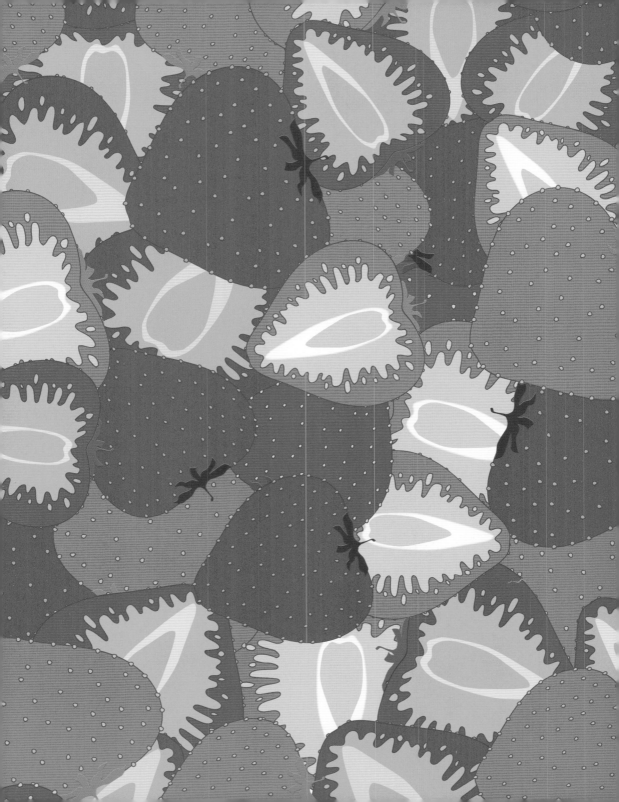

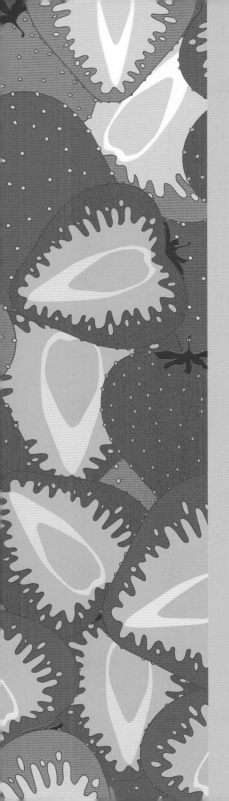

S

is for smoothies

Food is **fuel**. With the right ingredients inside you, your body can run at its best. Fresh juice is **packed with** all the most important elements: **vitamins**, **nutrients and minerals** which are **vital** for all kinds of chemical reactions that take place in our bodies every day. Smoothies often include **yogurt** to give the added dimension of a creamy texture. Made with the whole fruit, smoothies also provide plenty of fiber for that added nutritional value.

Oh so soothing

You gave it all in your workout,
now it's your turn to
get something back.
Just stretch out,
relax and imbibe.

pineapple pleasure

A great one for pineapple lovers, say
goodbye to your aches and pains with a hit
of these healthy nutrients.

¼ **pineapple, peeled and cut into chunks**
½ **banana**
½ **cup low-fat yogurt, frozen overnight,**
   or low-fat yogurt plus 4 ice cubes
¾ **cup frozen peeled pineapple**

How to do it Put the fresh pineapple
through an electric juicer. Pour the juice into
a blender or food processor, add all the
remaining ingredients and blend until smooth
and creamy. Serve immediately.

NUTRIENTS:
Packed with: vitamins
B5, B6, B7, C; calcium,
magnesium, phosphate,
manganese, potassium;
iodine
Plenty of: vitamins B1,
B3, B12, beta-carotene,
folic acid; zinc
Also contains: vitamin
E; copper, iron; fiber;
selenium

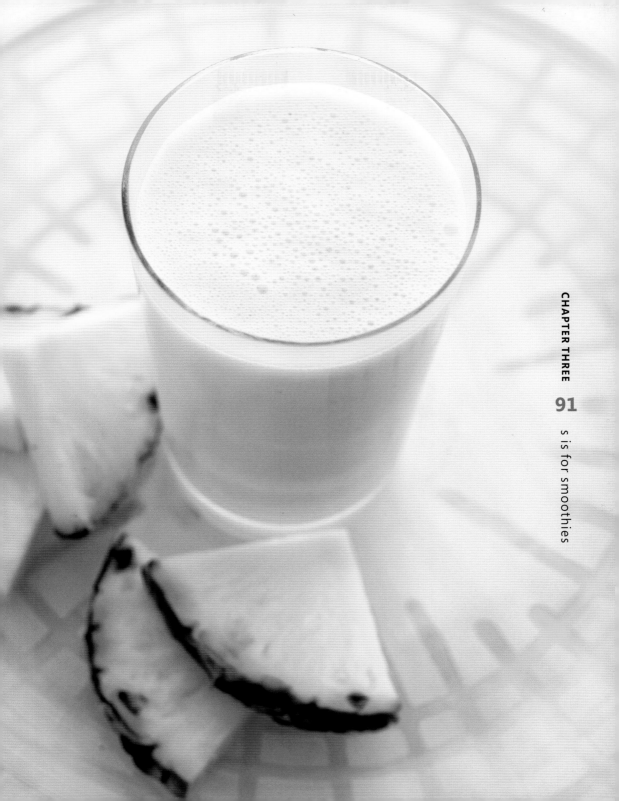

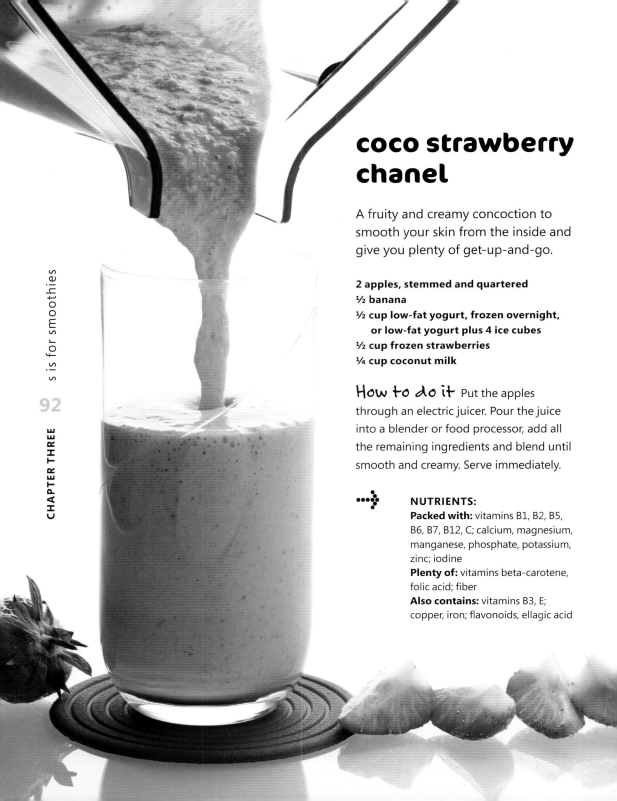

coco strawberry chanel

A fruity and creamy concoction to smooth your skin from the inside and give you plenty of get-up-and-go.

2 apples, stemmed and quartered
½ banana
½ cup low-fat yogurt, frozen overnight, or low-fat yogurt plus 4 ice cubes
½ cup frozen strawberries
¼ cup coconut milk

How to do it Put the apples through an electric juicer. Pour the juice into a blender or food processor, add all the remaining ingredients and blend until smooth and creamy. Serve immediately.

NUTRIENTS:
Packed with: vitamins B1, B2, B5, B6, B7, B12, C; calcium, magnesium, manganese, phosphate, potassium, zinc; iodine
Plenty of: vitamins beta-carotene, folic acid; fiber
Also contains: vitamins B3, E; copper, iron; flavonoids, ellagic acid

Kick off the day with one of these beauties!

papaya lime

For a cool wake-up call to boost your energy at breakfast, pop a slice of papaya in the freezer before you turn in, then you are good to go.

3 oranges, halved
¼ lime
½ banana
½ cup low-fat yogurt, frozen overnight, or low-fat yogurt plus 4 ice cubes
1 slice (1 inch thick) papaya, peeled, seeded and frozen overnight

How to do it Squeeze the juice from the oranges and the lime. Pour the juices into a blender or food processor, add all the remaining ingredients and blend until smooth and creamy. Serve immediately.

> **NUTRIENTS:**
> **Packed with:** vitamins B1, B2, B6, B7, B12, C, beta-carotene; calcium, magnesium, manganese, phosphate, potassium, zinc; iodine
> **Plenty of:** vitamins B5, folic acid; iron; fiber
> **Also contains:** vitamin E; copper; flavonoids, limonene

breakfast burner

Superfood blueberries to stimulate your brain combine with a smooth selection of ingredients to settle your digestion and give you energy for the rest of the morning.

3 oranges, halved
2 pieces (about 1-inch cubes) peeled pineapple
½ banana
½ cup low-fat yogurt, frozen overnight, or low-fat yogurt plus 4 ice cubes
¼ cup blueberries
½ mango, peeled and pitted

How to do it Squeeze the juice from the oranges. Pour the juice into a blender or food processor, add all the remaining ingredients and blend until smooth and creamy. Serve immediately.

> **NUTRIENTS:**
> **Packed with:** vitamins B1, B2, B5, B6, B7, B12, C, beta-carotene; calcium, copper, magnesium, manganese, phosphate, potassium, zinc, fiber; flavonoids, iodine
> **Plenty of:** vitamins B3, E, folic acid; iron
> **Also contains:** ellagic acid

maui baby smoothie

There's almost nothing missing from this great smoothie—a brilliant breakfast drink to get you ready for the day. Or try one as your lunchtime boost, especially if you are watching your weight. It'll keep you going all day long.

¼ pineapple, peeled and cut into chunks
½ banana
½ cup low-fat yogurt, frozen overnight, or low-fat yogurt plus 4 ice cubes
½ slice (1 inch thick) papaya, peeled, seeded and frozen overnight
½ mango, peeled and pitted
10 strawberries
2 tablespoons coconut milk

How to do it Put the pineapple through an electric juicer. Pour the juice into a blender or food processor, add all the remaining ingredients and blend until smooth and creamy. Serve immediately.

 NUTRIENTS:
Packed with: vitamins B complex, C, beta-carotene; potassium
Plenty of: copper, manganese
Also contains: ellagic acid, flavonoids

tropavado

Cholesterol-lowering avocado lends a smooth texture to this smoothie, which also offers the energizing zing of freshly squeezed orange juice.

3 oranges, halved
½ avocado, peeled and pitted
½ mango, peeled and pitted

How to do it Squeeze the juice from the oranges. Pour the juice into a blender or food processor, add all the remaining ingredients and blend until smooth and creamy. Serve immediately.

 NUTRIENTS:
Packed with: vitamins B5, B6, C, E, beta-carotene; copper, potassium, manganese; fiber
Plenty of: vitamins B1, B2, folic acid; iron, magnesium, phosphate
Also contains: vitamin B7; calcium, zinc; flavonoids; iodine, limonene

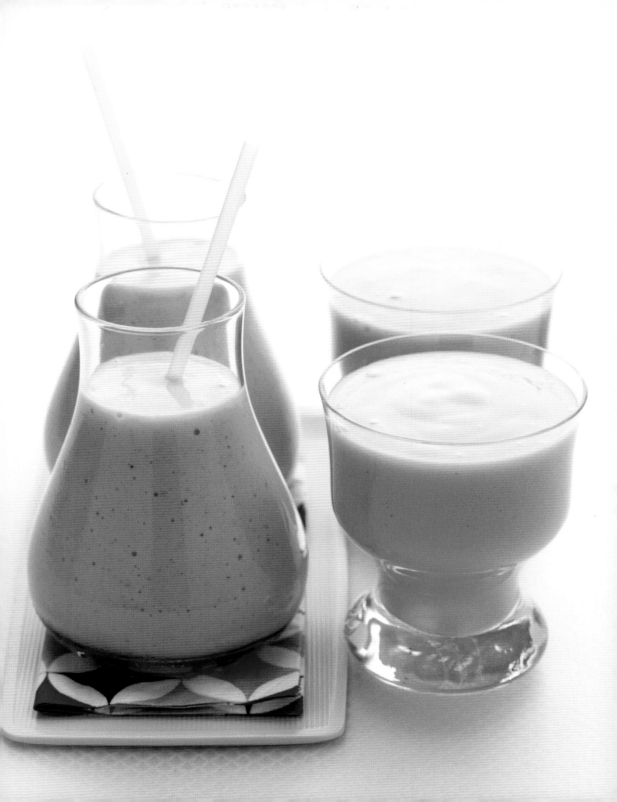

plant power phytonutrients

The prefix "phyto" comes from the Greek word for "plant," so the term phytonutrients simply means the good stuff found in juicy fruits and vegetables. You don't actually need these good guys to stay alive (like you do proteins, fats, vitamins and minerals), but if you want to keep your youthful complexion and energy, and help your body stay healthy, phytonutrients may be your new best friends.

Tell me more ...

In plants, phytonutrients are like an immune system, providing disease control, insecticide and sunscreen, as well as cleansing unwanted toxins that jeopardize optimum performance.

In humans, they can wage war on the enemies of your body—free radicals, cholesterol, and anything else that we don't want because they mean our bodies are not on top form.

Now for the science. What are some of these phytonutrients?

Carotenoids are found in red, orange and yellow foods. These big-hitters spark up your immune system and nurture your reproductive system.

Flavonoids boost the strength of blood vessels (because no one wants leaky veins).

Lignans cut cholesterol and can help keep you slim (that's good news!).

Phenols are the universal repairmen; they work to keep your cells in good shape.

Sulfides are all about physical flexibility—mind-bending!

Where do we get all that?

If you tend to get stuck in a rut, tossing the same old thing in the juicer every time, think again. Without variety, you don't have a hope of capturing the range of goodies available. Go out and fill your cart with new things: pears, guavas, kale, pumpkins ... they're all great. Go on! Be adventurous. It's the only way.

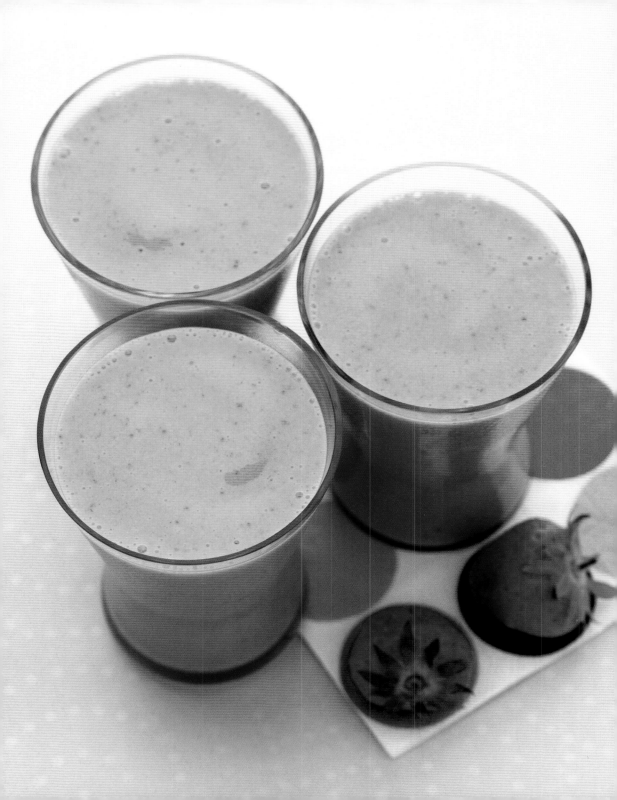

Need a cool, dairy-free smoothie?

If you don't eat dairy products, why not try substituting some soy yogurt instead of the regular yogurt?

strawberry cool

The ultimate indulgence, this tastes like the best strawberries and cream in a glass.

3 oranges, halved
1 banana
½ cup low-fat yogurt, frozen overnight, or low-fat yogurt plus 4 ice cubes
1 cup frozen strawberries

How to do it Squeeze the juice from the oranges. Pour the juice into a blender or food processor, add all the remaining ingredients and blend until smooth and creamy. Serve immediately.

NUTRIENTS:
Packed with: vitamins B2, B5, B6, B7, C, folic acid; calcium, magnesium, manganese, phosphate, potassium; iodine
Plenty of: vitamins B1, B12, beta-carotene; zinc,
Also contains: vitamins B3, E; copper, iron; ellagic acid, flavonoids; fiber; selenium

Breathe deeply

Because breathing properly is healthy, too, so make sure you really fill your lungs to top up with oxygen. Plus you can breathe in the light, flowery scent of lychees. Don't you just love it?

guava lychee smoothie

A great digestive aid, this subtle pink smoothie is a good lunchtime choice. Add a handful of strawberries if you cannot find guavas in your local store.

3 apples, stemmed and quartered
¼ guava, peeled
½ banana
½ cup low-fat yogurt, frozen overnight, or low-fat yogurt plus 4 ice cubes
5 canned lychees, frozen overnight

How to do it Put the apples and guava through an electric juicer. Pour the juice into a blender or food processor, add all the remaining ingredients and blend until smooth and creamy. Serve immediately.

NUTRIENTS:
Packed with: vitamins B1, B2, B5, B6, B7, B12, C, beta-carotene; calcium, copper, magnesium, manganese, phosphate, potassium, zinc; iodine
Plenty of: vitamins E, folic acid; fiber; flavonoids
Also contains: vitamin B3; iron

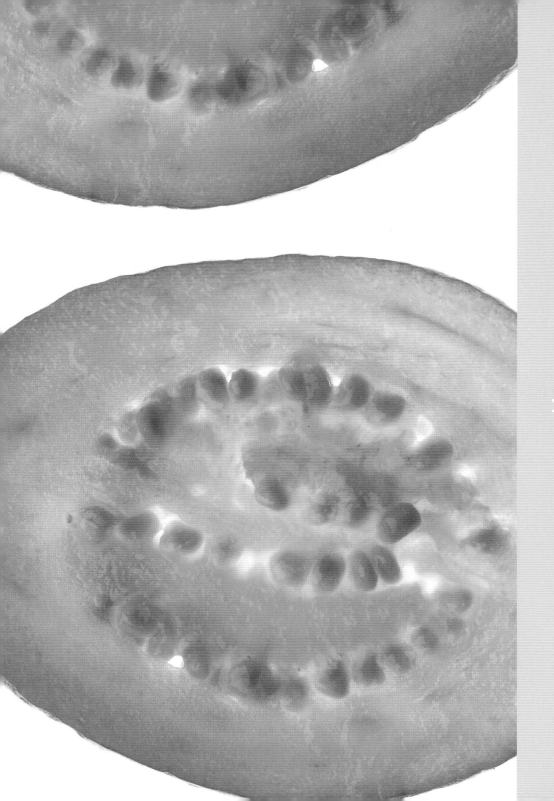

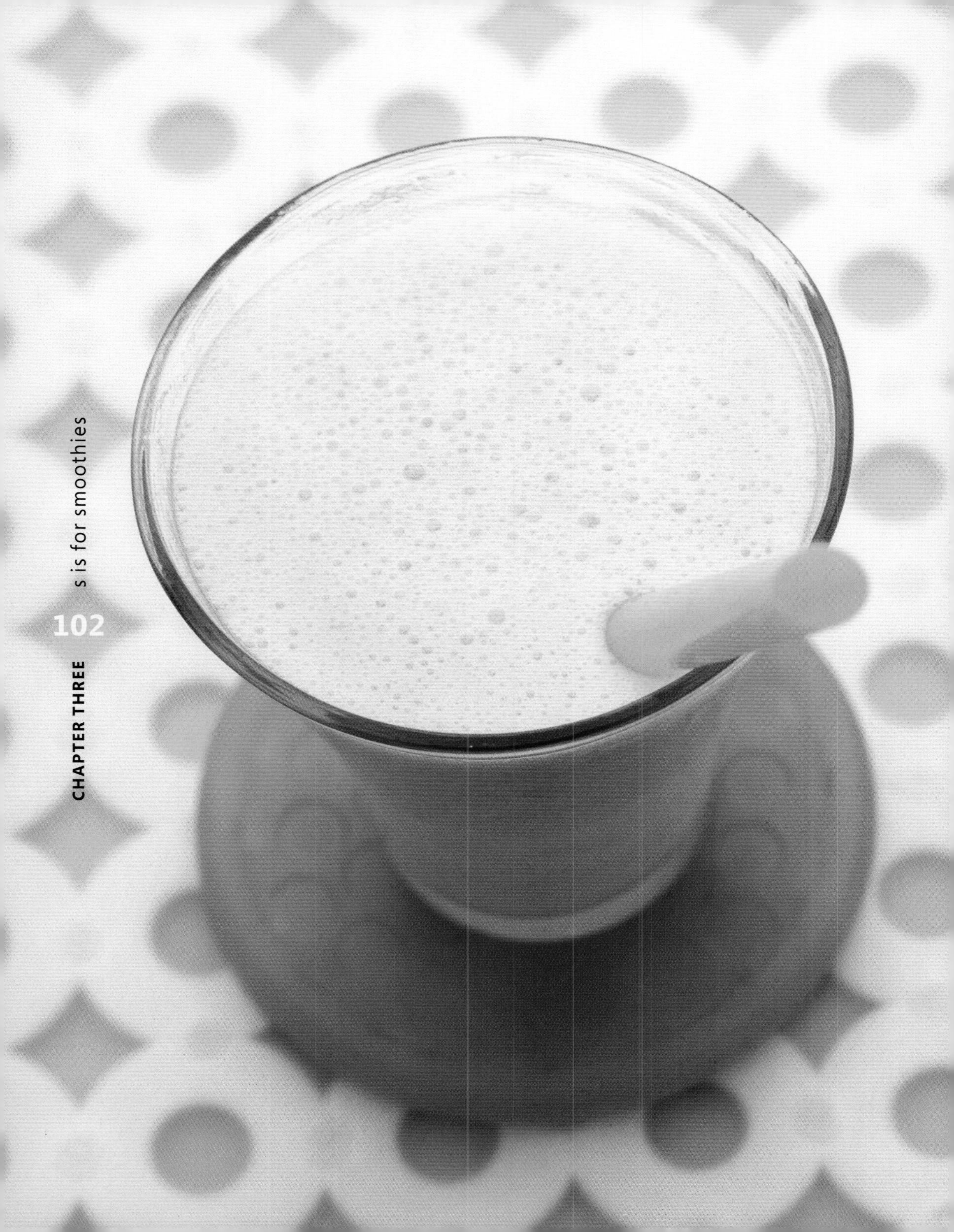

Enter the dragon

You'll get plenty of raw power from this health-giving juice made with longan fruit, also known as dragon eye fruit.

dragon eye smoothie

Longan fruit is called the dragon eye for its resemblance to that mythical creature. Tap into its power and energy with this cool and sophisticated smoothie. You can use canned lychees, frozen overnight, if you can't find longan fruit.

3 apples, stemmed and quartered
½ banana
½ cup low-fat yogurt, frozen overnight, or low-fat yogurt plus 4 ice cubes
12 longan fruit, peeled, pitted and frozen overnight

How to do it Put the apples through an electric juicer. Pour the juice into a blender or food processor, add all the remaining ingredients and blend until smooth and creamy. Serve immediately.

NUTRIENTS:
Packed with: vitamins B1, B2, B5, B6, B7, C; calcium, copper, magnesium, manganese, phosphate, potassium, zinc; iodine
Plenty of: beta-carotene, folic acid; iron; fiber
Also contains: vitamins B3, E; flavonoids

papaya paradise

A warm and sunny juice blend to make you feel great all day—get a taste of paradise into your life.

3 oranges, halved
½ banana
½ cup low-fat yogurt, frozen overnight, or low-fat yogurt plus 4 ice cubes
½ slice (1 inch thick) papaya, peeled, seeded and frozen overnight
½ cup frozen strawberries

How to do it Squeeze the juice from the oranges. Pour the juice into a blender or food processor, add all the remaining ingredients and blend until smooth and creamy. Serve immediately.

NUTRIENTS:
Packed with: vitamins B1, B2, B5, B6, B7, B12, C, beta-carotene, folic acid; calcium, magnesium, manganese, phosphate, potassium, zinc; iodine
Plenty of: vitamin B3; iron
Also contains: vitamin E; copper; fiber; ellagic acid, flavonoids

mangosteen apricot

With a superboost for your immune system, seek out mangosteens from your local Thai or Asian store. You can substitute five canned lychees, frozen overnight, if you can't find mangosteens.

3 apples, stemmed and quartered
3 mangosteens, peeled, pitted and frozen overnight
½ banana
½ cup low-fat yogurt, frozen overnight, or low-fat yogurt plus 4 ice cubes
2 apricots, pitted

How to do it Put the apples through an electric juicer. Pour the juice into a blender or food processor, add all the remaining ingredients and blend until smooth and creamy. Serve immediately.

NUTRIENTS:
Packed with: vitamins B1, B2, B5, B6, B7, B12, C, beta-carotene; calcium, magnesium, manganese, phosphate, potassium, zinc; iodine
Plenty of: folic acid; copper; fiber
Also contains: vitamins B3, E; iron; flavonoids

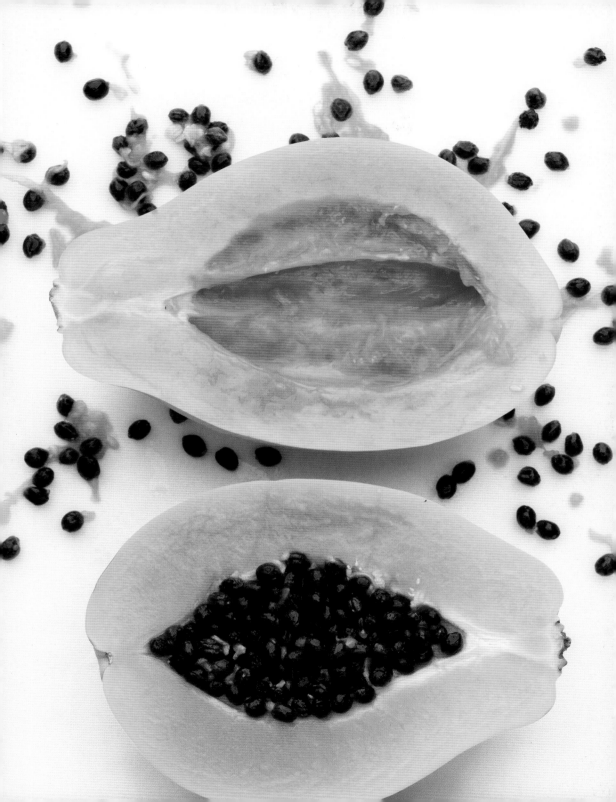

cherry nice

There's no doubt that this cherry nice smoothie is packed with nutrients to make you cherry healthy.

4 apples, stemmed and quartered
¼ pineapple, peeled and cut into chunks
2 thin slices ginger root
½ cup cherries, pitted
2 tablespoons coconut milk

How to do it Put the apples, pineapple and ginger through an electric juicer. Pour the juice into a blender or food processor, add all the remaining ingredients and blend until smooth. Serve immediately.

NUTRIENTS:
Packed with: vitamins B1, B5, B6, B7, C; copper, manganese, potassium
Plenty of: vitamin B2, folic acid; omega-3
Also contains: iron

figamajig

A treat for your digestive tract, Figamajig will work its magic through your system, smoothing out problems along the way. Just remember to soak the prunes the night before. You can use any kind of figs for this smoothie.

2 apples, stemmed and quartered
½ banana
½ cup low-fat yogurt, frozen overnight, or low-fat yogurt plus 4 ice cubes
¼ cup blackberries
2 black figs
5 prunes, pitted and soaked overnight in cold water, then drained

How to do it Put the apples through an electric juicer. Pour the juice into a blender or food processor, add all the remaining ingredients and blend until smooth and creamy. Serve immediately.

NUTRIENTS:
Packed with: vitamins B1, B2, B5, B6, B7, B12, C, beta-carotene, folic acid; calcium, copper, iron, magnesium, manganese, phosphate, potassium, zinc; fiber; iodine
Plenty of: vitamins B3, E
Also contains: ellagic acid, flavonoids

papaya passion

Here's a shot of energy to get you on track, and slow-burning endurance to keep you going.

3 oranges, halved
½ banana
½ cup low-fat yogurt, frozen overnight,
  or low-fat yogurt plus 4 ice cubes
½ slice (1 inch thick) papaya, peeled,
  seeded and frozen overnight
2 pieces (about 2-inch cubes) peeled
  pineapple
½ passionfruit, pulp scooped out

How to do it Squeeze the juice from the oranges. Pour the juice into a blender or food processor, add all the remaining ingredients and blend until smooth and creamy. Serve immediately.

NUTRIENTS:
Packed with: vitamins B1, B2, B5, B6, B7, B12, C, beta-carotene; calcium, magnesium, manganese, phosphate, potassium, zinc; iodine
Plenty of: vitamins B3, folic acid; copper, iron
Also contains: vitamin E; fiber; flavonoids

raspberry gold

Raspberries are healing and soothing and in this smoothie—with a team of nutrient-rich fruits in support—they bring your digestive system up to the gold-standard.

3 apples, stemmed and quartered
2 pieces (about 2-inch cubes) frozen peeled
  pineapple
½ banana
½ cup low-fat yogurt, frozen overnight,
  or low-fat yogurt plus 4 ice cubes
1¼ cups frozen raspberries

How to do it Put the apples and pineapple through an electric juicer. Pour the juices into a blender or food processor, add all the remaining ingredients and blend until smooth and creamy. Serve immediately.

NUTRIENTS:
Packed with: vitamins B1, B2, B5, B6, B7, B12, C, beta-carotene, folic acid; calcium, copper, magnesium, manganese, phosphate, potassium, zinc; fiber; iodine, flavonoids, ellagic acid
Plenty of: vitamins B3, E; iron

Don't wait till summer comes

Don't miss out!
Freeze your summer fruits when they are in season so you can enjoy them all through the winter months.

six-fruit smoothie

A rainbow of fruit colors for a spectrum of nutrients to improve your circulation and get your immune system in great shape.

3 oranges, halved
½ banana
½ cup low-fat yogurt, frozen overnight, or low-fat yogurt plus 4 ice cubes
7 frozen strawberries
¼ cup frozen raspberries
¼ cup frozen blueberries
½ passionfruit, pulp scooped out

How to do it Squeeze the juice from the oranges. Pour the juice into a blender or food processor, add all the remaining ingredients and blend until smooth and creamy. Serve immediately.

NUTRIENTS:
Packed with: vitamins B1, B2, B3, B5, B6, B7, B12, C, beta-carotene, folic acid; calcium, copper; fiber; ellagic acid, flavonoids, iodine
Plenty of: vitamin E; iron, magnesium, manganese, phosphate, potassium, zinc

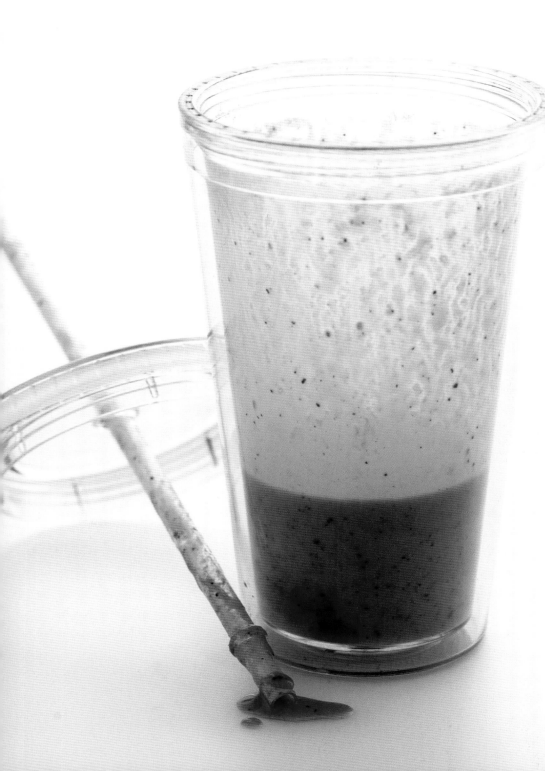

slim with juices

Imagine a world in which dieting is filled with such deliciousness that you can barely wait to begin. It's not a dream—you can make it a reality. And this weight-loss regime won't leave you feeling tired and flat. So what are you waiting for? Let's get juicing! And if you crave a little sweet creaminess, add a banana and a little low-fat yogurt to your smoothie. Silky-smooth and fabulously filling, you won't feel like you're dieting at all.

Does it speed up metabolism?

Not all by itself, no. You're not going to get out of exercising that easily! But leafy greens, blueberries and other fruits, whole grains and plenty of fiber certainly help. If you can, have a hearty breakfast and choose to replace either lunch or dinner with one of our special smoothies.

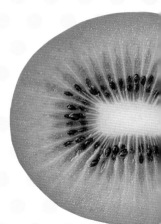

What do we need?

Very little. It's a simple process.

First, gather the weight-loss fruit basket: acai berries, apples, avocados, blackberries, blackcurrants, blueberries, carrots, coconuts, fennel, kiwis, mangosteens, oranges, passionfruit, peaches, pears, prunes, raspberries, spinach, starfruit, strawberries, watermelons.

Once a day, blend some of these with cow milk, soy milk or low-fat yogurt for a filling smoothie that replaces just one of your usual meals.

Then all you need to do is drink in the weight-loss nutrients.

- **B-vitamins**—pump up the metabolism and burn the fat.

- **Vitamin C**—burns the sugar, stores the iron.

- **Calcium**—a well-known slimmer's friend that's good for strong bones, too.

- **Iron**—gives an energy-boost for efficient weight loss.

- **Fiber**—cranks up your digestive system.

- **Protein**—keeps hunger at bay.

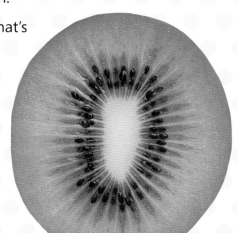

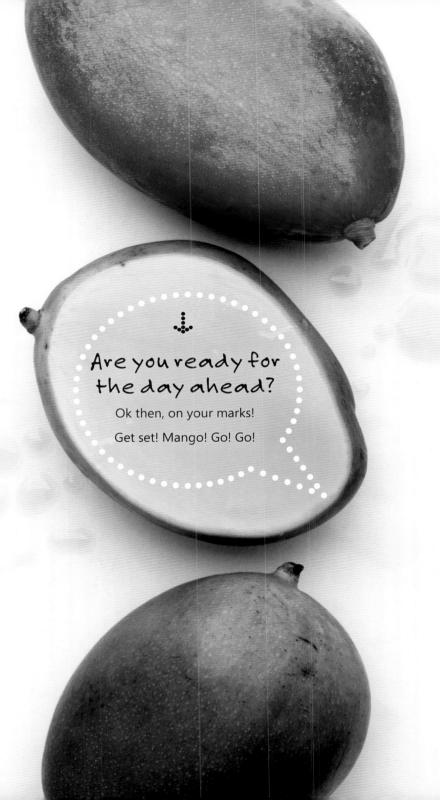

Are you ready for
the day ahead?

Ok then, on your marks!

Get set! Mango! Go! Go!

mango madness

Exotic, delicious and soothing, choose mango to keep your digestive system in good working order with banana for well-functioning nerves and high energy levels.

3 oranges, halved
½ banana
½ cup low-fat yogurt, frozen overnight,
 or low-fat yogurt plus 4 ice cubes
1½ mangoes, peeled and pitted

How to do it
Squeeze the juice from the oranges. Pour the juice into a blender or food processor, add all the remaining ingredients and blend until smooth and creamy. Serve immediately.

> **NUTRIENTS:**
> **Packed with:** vitamins B1, B2, B5, B6, B7, B12, C, beta-carotene; calcium, copper, magnesium, manganese, phosphate, potassium, zinc; fiber; iodine
> **Plenty of:** vitamins B3, E, folic acid; iron
> **Also contains:** flavonoids

forbidden fruit smoothie

If the rules forbid this packed-with-goodness combo—break them! But why should they? This beautiful pink smoothie has something for everything and will give your body and brain a boost.

3 apples, stemmed and quartered
½ banana
½ cup low-fat yogurt, frozen overnight,
 or low-fat yogurt plus 4 ice cubes
10 cherries, pitted
¼ cup frozen raspberries
7 frozen strawberries
½ peach, pitted

How to do it
Put the apples through an electric juicer. Pour the juice into a blender or food processor, add all the remaining ingredients and blend until smooth and creamy. Serve immediately.

> **NUTRIENTS:**
> **Packed with:** vitamins B1, B2, B3, B5, B6, B7, B12, C, beta-carotene, folic acid; calcium, copper, magnesium, manganese, phosphate, potassium, zinc; fiber; ellagic acid, flavonoids, iodine
> **Plenty of:** iron
> **Also contains:** vitamin E

acai berry fiesta

A positive fiesta of nutrients burst out of this energy-promoting smoothie, full of antioxidants to chase down and destroy toxins in your system.

3 apples, stemmed and quartered
½ banana
½ cup low-fat yogurt, frozen overnight,
    or low-fat yogurt plus 4 ice cubes
2¼ ounces frozen acai puree
¼ cup frozen blueberries
7 frozen strawberries

How to do it Put the apples through an electric juicer. Pour the juice into a blender or food processor, add all the remaining ingredients and blend until smooth and creamy. Serve immediately.

NUTRIENTS:
Packed with: vitamins B1, B2, B5, B6, B7, B12, C, E, beta-carotene, folic acid, calcium, iron, magnesium, manganese, phosphate, potassium, zinc; fiber; iodine
Plenty of: vitamins B3; copper; ellagic acid, flavonoids

banana nut-arama

With slow-release energy to keep you going and soothing qualities for your digestive system, this smoothie has just a hint of sweetness from a spoonful of honey.

generous ⅓ cup soy milk
1½ bananas
½ cup soy yogurt, frozen overnight,
    or soy yogurt plus 4 ice cubes
2 teaspoons chopped almonds
1 teaspoon chopped walnuts
1 teaspoon honey
3 ice cubes

How to do it Put all the ingredients in a blender or food processor and blend until smooth and creamy.
Serve immediately.

NUTRIENTS:
Packed with: vitamins B2, B5, B6, B7, B12, C; calcium, magnesium, manganese, phosphate, potassium, zinc; iodine
Plenty of: vitamins B1, E, folic acid; copper
Also contains: vitamin B3, beta-carotene; iron; fiber; selenium

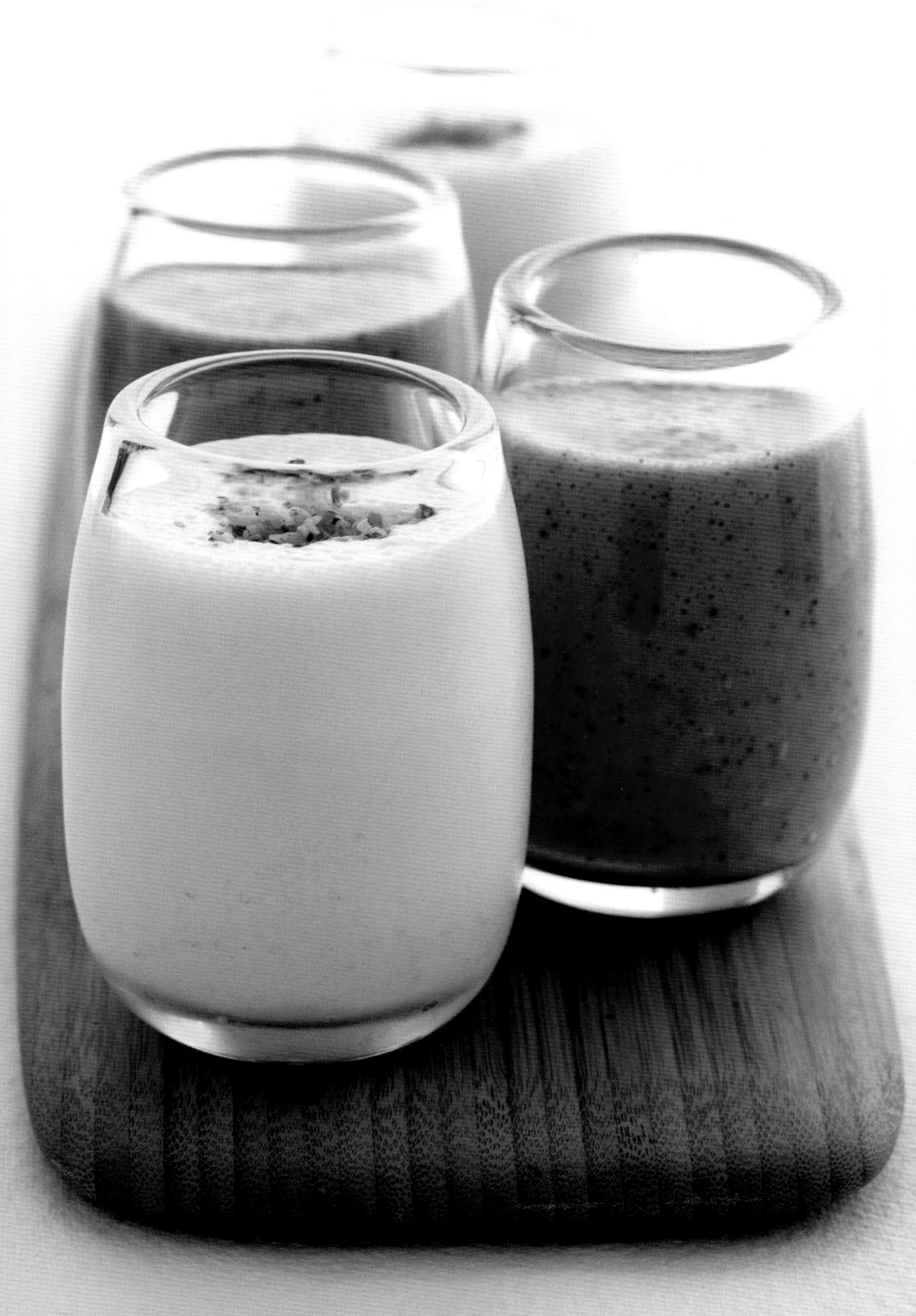

CHAPTER THREE

s is for smoothies

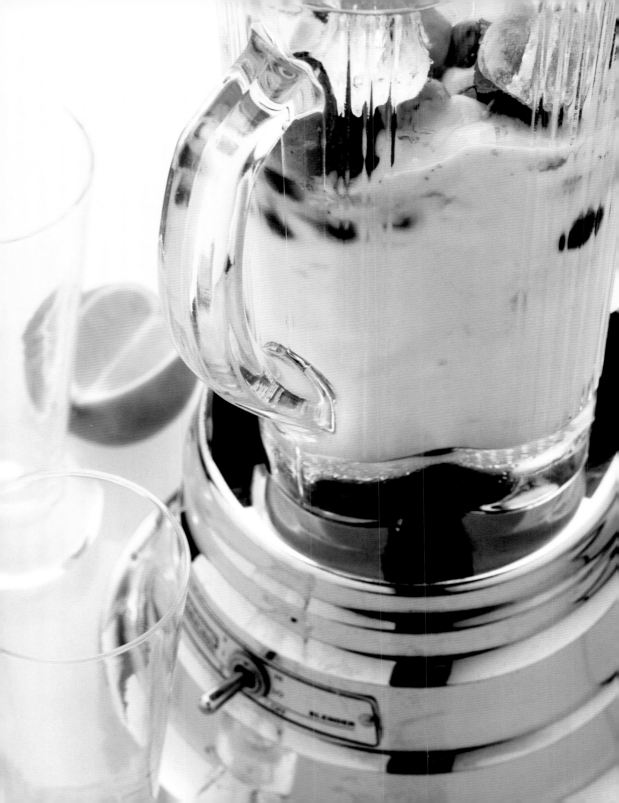

blueberry coco-lime

Packed with superfoods, this creamy concoction is a tropical superboost.

¼ lime
⅔ cup soy milk
½ banana
½ cup soy yogurt, frozen overnight,
    or soy yogurt plus 4 ice cubes
¼ cup frozen blueberries
¼ cup coconut milk
3 mint leaves

How to do it Squeeze the juice from the lime. Pour the juice into a blender or food processor, add all the remaining ingredients and blend until smooth and the mint leaves are finely chopped. (Alternatively, you can simply chop the mint leaves and add them to the juice.) Serve immediately.

> **NUTRIENTS:**
> **Packed with:** vitamin C; copper, manganese, phosphate, potassium; fiber
> **Plenty of:** vitamins B1, B2, B6, B7, E, beta-carotene; calcium, iron, magnesium; selenium
> **Also contains:** vitamins B3, B5, folic acid; zinc; ellagic acid, flavonoids, iodine, isoflavones

hot apple & cardamom prune

With apples to remove impurities and bananas to promote healthy nerve function and control blood pressure, this is a great lunchtime smoothie.

6 apples, stemmed and quartered
½ banana
½ cup low-fat yogurt, frozen overnight,
    or low-fat yogurt plus 4 ice cubes
6 prunes, pitted and soaked overnight in
    cold water, then drained
seeds from 3 cardamom pods

How to do it Peel, core and chop 3 of the apples, put in a pan with 1 tablespoon water, bring to a boil, then simmer for 5 minutes until pulpy. (Alternatively, use ¾ cup applesauce.) Put the remaining apples through an electric juicer. Pour the juice into a blender or food processor, add the stewed apples and all the remaining ingredients and blend until smooth and creamy. Warm the smoothie in a pan over low heat and serve immediately.

> **NUTRIENTS:**
> **Packed with:** vitamins B2, B5, B6, B7, C; calcium, magnesium, manganese, phosphate, potassium; fiber; iodine
> **Plenty of:** vitamins B1, B12, folic acid; copper, iron, zinc
> **Also contains:** vitamins E, beta-carotene; selenium

Get in shape

If you need a bit of a nudge to get you started, here's a juice with a subtle kick of chili that is sure to get you off the starting blocks and away.

sporty spicy

If Sporty Spice were a smoothie, this is what she would be! The great taste of ripe mango combines fabulously with the spicy kick of chilies—while the yogurt takes the edge off.

3 oranges, halved
¼ lime
½ banana
½ cup low-fat yogurt, frozen overnight,
    or low-fat yogurt plus 4 ice cubes
1 mango, peeled and pitted
¼ chili (or to taste)

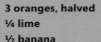 **How to do it** Squeeze the juice from the oranges and lime. Pour the juices into a blender or food processor, add all the remaining ingredients and blend until smooth and creamy. Serve immediately.

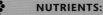

NUTRIENTS:
Packed with: vitamins B1, B2, B5, B6, B7, C, beta-carotene; calcium, copper, magnesium, manganese, phosphate, potassium, zinc; fiber; iodine
Plenty of: vitamins B12, E, folic acid; iron
Also contains: flavonoids; limonene

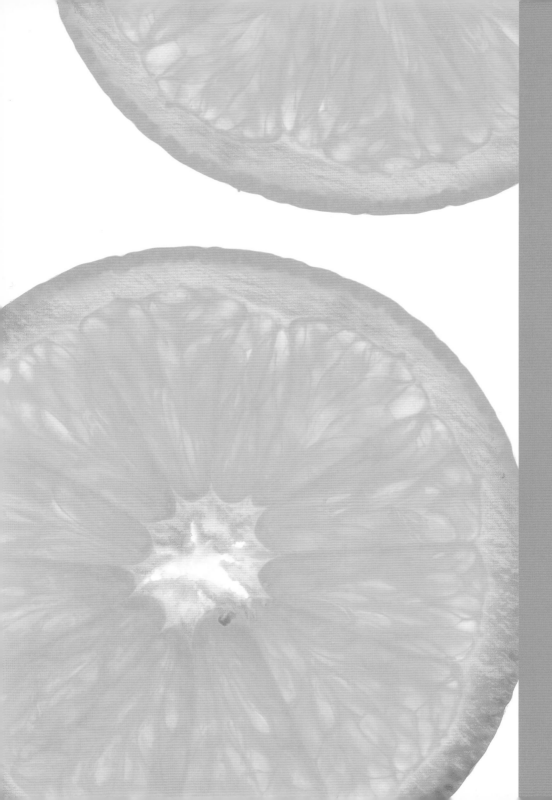

CHAPTER THREE

119

s is for smoothies

sunny-side up tropical fruits

Pure sunshine in a glass, from bananas to passionfruit and pineapples to mangoes, tropical fruits transport us beyond the office, the kitchen or the playroom and into a world where the sand is beneath our feet and the ocean laps at the shore. It's all about bringing a little bit of paradise to your day. Apart from that, tropical fruits bring a good dose of vital nutrients with them, too.

Tell me more …

All tropical fruits are low in fat, low in protein and high in carbs. What else you get depends entirely on your chosen tipple. If you're aiming for low-calorie but high vitamin C and folate, opt for something with a good squeeze of papaya. A juice made using pineapple will give you loads of vitamin C, but also high levels of manganese and copper. If you're after a happy pill, try something containing banana—its high levels of vitamin B6 help convert the amino acid tryptophan to serotonin, the ultimate feel-good hormone.

What will all that do for me?

- **Give you strength, focus, energy**—high levels of potassium in bananas keep you calm, while practically citrus-levels of vitamin C in the other tropical fruits keep your circulation pumping.

- **Make you super-elastic**—high levels of copper in pineapples and mangoes make tropical fruits a winning choice if you want to keep your joints supple (and copper fights off the signs of aging, too).

- **Provide heavyweight security**—many tropical fruits (including mangoes, papayas and guavas) are bursting with carotenoids. These are like heavyweight security that protect against attacks on your health.

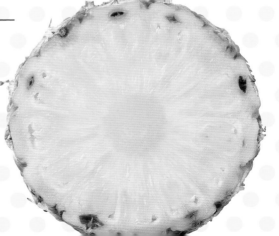

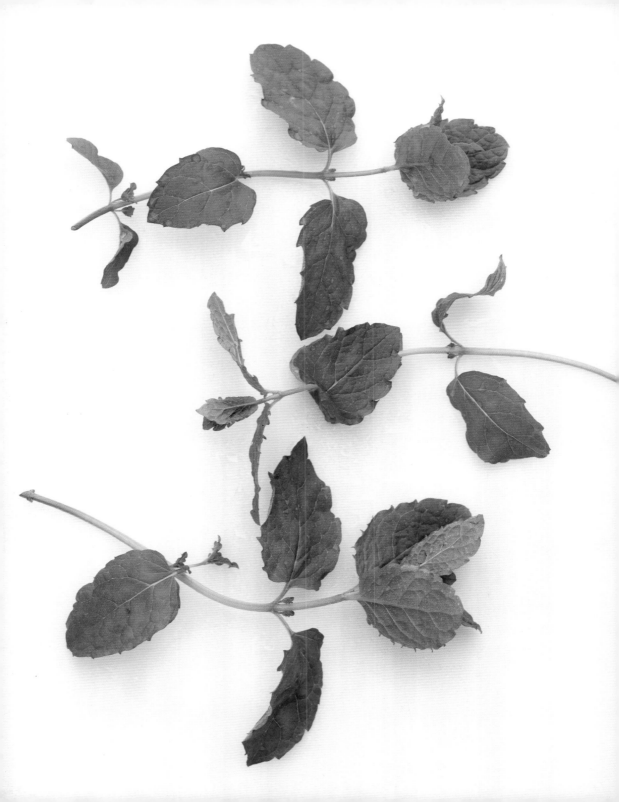

mintavado

Fresh with mint leaves and lime, the perfect counterbalance to the richness and creamy texture of the banana, yogurt and avocado.

¼ lime
⅔ cup soy milk
½ banana
½ cup soy yogurt, frozen overnight,
    or soy yogurt plus 4 ice cubes
½ avocado, peeled and pitted
3 mint leaves

How to do it Squeeze the juice from the lime. Pour the juice into a blender or food processor, add all the remaining ingredients and blend until smooth and the mint leaves are finely chopped. (Alternatively, you can simply chop the mint leaves and add them to the smoothie.) Serve immediately.

NUTRIENTS:
Packed with: vitamins B1, B2, B5, B6, B7, B12, C; calcium, magnesium, phosphate, potassium, zinc; iodine
Plenty of: vitamins B3, E, beta-carotene, folic acid; copper, manganese; fiber
Also contains: iron

kiwi banana smoothie

With a hit of those vital antioxidants along with heart-boosting nutrients, the best way to get all the benefits from kiwi is to blend it and drink it.

¼ pineapple, peeled and cut into chunks
½ lime
½ banana
½ cup low-fat yogurt, frozen overnight,
    or low-fat yogurt plus 4 ice cubes
1½ kiwis, peeled and halved

How to do it Put the pineapple through an electric juicer. Squeeze the juice from the lime. Pour the juices into a blender or food processor, add all the remaining ingredients and blend until smooth and creamy. Serve immediately.

NUTRIENTS:
Packed with: vitamins B1, B2, B5, B6, B7, B12, C, beta-carotene; calcium, copper, magnesium, manganese, phosphate, potassium, zinc; iodine
Plenty of: vitamins B3, folic acid
Also contains: vitamin E; iron; fiber

strawberries & peach summer smoothie

Whatever the weather is doing outside, you can be sure you'll feel the warm glow of summer when you try this sunshine-filled glass. From the orange of sunrise to the pink of sunset, the health boost will last all day.

¼ pineapple, peeled and cut into chunks
½ banana
½ cup low-fat yogurt, frozen overnight, or low-fat yogurt plus 4 ice cubes
10 frozen strawberries
1 peach, pitted

How to do it Put the pineapple through an electric juicer. Pour the juice into a blender or food processor, add all the remaining ingredients and blend until smooth and creamy. Serve immediately.

NUTRIENTS:
Packed with: vitamins B1, B2, B5, B6, B7, B12, C, beta-carotene, folic acid; calcium, copper, magnesium, manganese, phosphate, potassium, zinc; iodine
Plenty of: vitamin B3; iron
Also contains: vitamin E; fiber; ellagic acid, flavonoids

tart start

Blueberries make any smoothie a super-smoothie with their brain-boosting nutrients, and cranberries are not far behind, ensuring your heart keeps pace with your head.

3 apples, stemmed and quartered
½ banana
½ cup low-fat yogurt, frozen overnight, or low-fat yogurt plus 4 ice cubes
⅓ cup frozen cranberries
⅓ cup frozen blueberries

How to do it Put the apples through an electric juicer. Pour the juice into a blender or food processor, add all the remaining ingredients and blend until smooth and creamy. Serve immediately.

NUTRIENTS:
Packed with: vitamins B1, B2, B5, B6, B7, C, beta-carotene; calcium, magnesium, manganese, phosphate, potassium, zinc; iodine
Plenty of: vitamins E, folic acid; copper, iron; fiber
Also contains: vitamin B3; ellagic acid, flavonoids

cantaloupe & lychee smoothie

Even out the ups and downs of the day with a lunchtime smoothie that brings you slow-release energy packaged with calming nutrients to lower your blood pressure. It's just what you need when you have a busy afternoon at the office ahead of you.

3 apples, stemmed and quartered
½ banana
½ cup low-fat yogurt, frozen overnight, or low-fat yogurt plus 4 ice cubes
1 slice (1 inch thick) peeled cantaloupe melon, frozen overnight
5 canned lychees, frozen overnight

How to do it Put the apples through an electric juicer. Pour the juice into a blender or food processor, add all the remaining ingredients and blend until smooth and creamy. Serve immediately.

NUTRIENTS:
Packed with: vitamins B1, B2, B5, B6, B7, B12, C, beta-carotene; calcium, copper, magnesium, manganese, phosphate, potassium, zinc; iodine
Plenty of: folic acid
Also contains: vitamins B3, E; iron; fiber; flavonoids

strawberry soy smoothie

Do something simply and do it well. Here's a classic example of that wise old saying.

⅔ cup soy milk
½ banana
½ cup soy yogurt, frozen overnight, or soy yogurt plus 4 ice cubes
¾ cup strawberries

How to do it Put all the ingredients in a blender or food processor and blend until smooth and creamy. Serve immediately.

NUTRIENTS:
Packed with: vitamins A, C, folic acid; calcium, magnesium, manganese, phosphate, potassium
Plenty of: vitamins B1, B6, K; copper
Also contains: vitamins B3, B5; fiber; selenium

Perfection in a glass

Flat or round, yellow flesh or white —they're all peachy perfect when it comes to smoothies!

peachy roast smoothie

Broiling the peaches gives a whole new dimension of flavor, not to mention a burst of nutrients. One for the fitness fans, this is great for easing your muscles when you've had a mega-dose of exercise.

2 peaches, halved and pitted
¼ pineapple, peeled and cut into chunks
½ banana
½ cup low-fat yogurt, frozen overnight,
    or low-fat yogurt plus 4 ice cubes
3 ice cubes

How to do it Broil the peaches under a hot broiler about 5 minutes until caramelized. Put in the freezer and leave 15 to 30 minutes until chilled. Put the pineapple through an electric juicer. Pour the juice into a blender or food processor, add all the remaining ingredients, including the broiled peaches, and blend until smooth and creamy. Serve immediately.

NUTRIENTS:
Packed with: vitamins B1, B2, B5, B6, B7, C, beta-carotene; calcium, copper, magnesium, manganese, phosphate, potassium, zinc; iodine
Plenty of: vitamin B3, folic acid; fiber
Also contains: vitamin E; iron

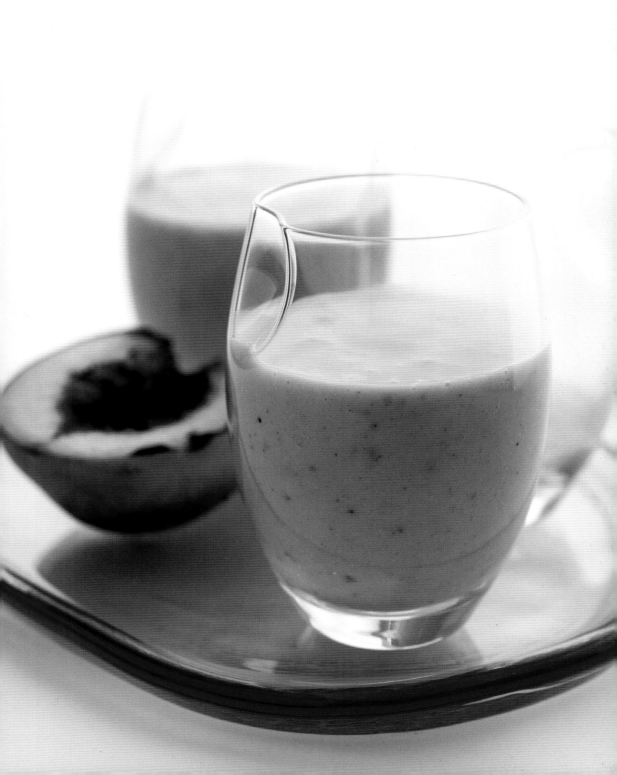

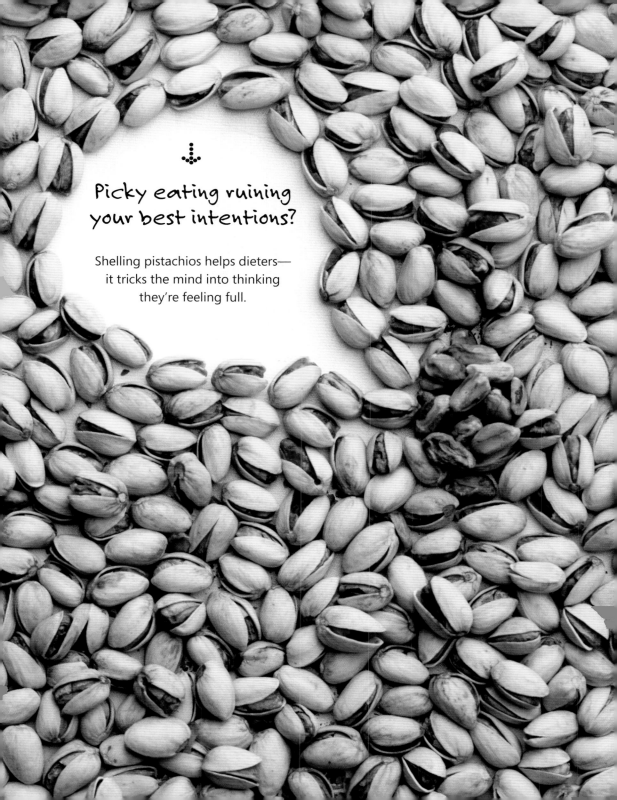

Picky eating ruining your best intentions?

Shelling pistachios helps dieters—
it tricks the mind into thinking
they're feeling full.

pistachio cacao smoothie

Make your own almond milk to use in this delicious smoothie.

1⅔ cups almonds
2 teaspoons honey (optional)
1½ bananas, halved
1 cup low-fat yogurt, frozen overnight, or low-fat yogurt plus 4 ice cubes
2 tablespoons shelled pistachio nuts
1 teaspoon cacao nibs
3 ice cubes

How to do it To make the almond milk, soak the almonds in water overnight, then drain. Blend them with 4 cups fresh water, adding a little of the honey, if you wish. Strain through a fine cheesecloth-lined strainer, squeezing the pulp to create as much almond milk as you can. (Alternatively, use ready-made almond milk.) Put a generous ⅓ cup almond milk into a blender or food processor, add all the remaining ingredients and blend until smooth and creamy. Serve immediately.

NUTRIENTS:
Packed with: vitamins B1, B2, B5, B6, B7, B12, C, beta-carotene, folic acid; calcium, copper, magnesium, manganese, phosphate, potassium, zinc; iodine
Plenty of: vitamins B3, E; iron; fiber
Also contains: selenium

pecan caramello smoothie

A super-smooth smoothie, sweet and creamy, you'll absorb a long energy burst with this banana-rich cocktail to keep you going through the day.

generous ⅓ cup soy milk
1½ bananas, halved
1 cup soy yogurt, frozen overnight, or soy yogurt plus 4 ice cubes
2 tablespoons chopped pecans
3 tablespoons caramel syrup
1 teaspoon honey
3 ice cubes

How to do it Put all the ingredients in a blender or food processor and blend until smooth and creamy. Serve immediately.

NUTRIENTS:
Packed with: vitamins B1, B2, B5, B6, B7, B12, C, folic acid; calcium, copper, magnesium, manganese, phosphate, potassium, zinc; iodine
Plenty of: vitamins B3, E, beta-carotene; iron; fiber
Also contains: selenium

The athletes' tipple

You just can't **beet** the red juice for helping build the stamina for long-distance racing. So why don't you try this intense smoothie, and you could be the red-hot favourite.

red velvet smoothie

The natural boost of beet juice increases the flow of oxygen around your body, so whatever activities you are indulging in—from Olympic sports to running for the bus—this is a great way to start your day.

1 beet, cut into chunks
½ banana
1 cup low-fat yogurt, frozen overnight, or low-fat yogurt plus 4 ice cubes
¾ cup cup cherries, pitted

How to do it Put the beet through an electric juicer. Pour the juice into a blender or food processor, add all the remaining ingredients and blend until smooth and creamy. Serve immediately.

NUTRIENTS:
Packed with: vitamins B2, B5, B6, B7, B12, C, beta-carotene, folic acid; calcium, magnesium, manganese, phosphate, potassium, zinc; iodine
Plenty of: vitamin B1; copper
Also contains: vitamins B3, E; iron; fiber; flavonoids

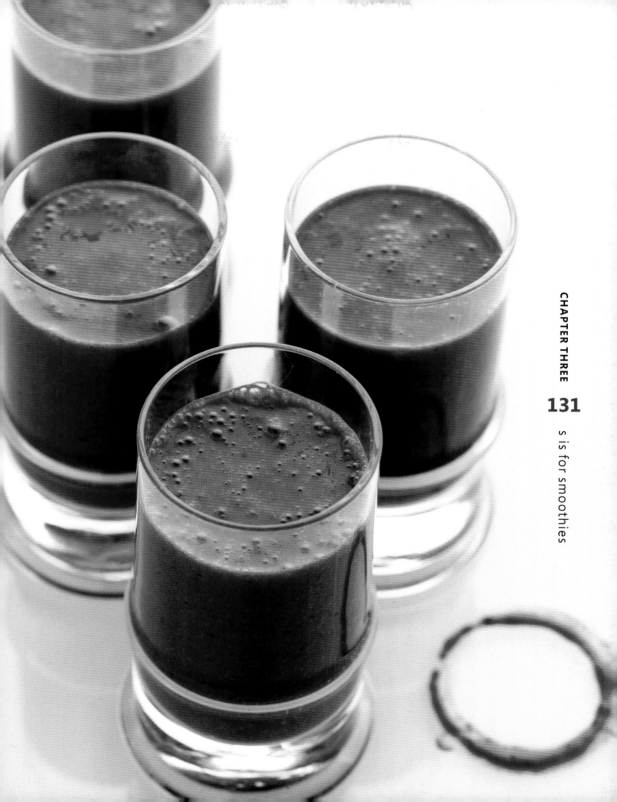

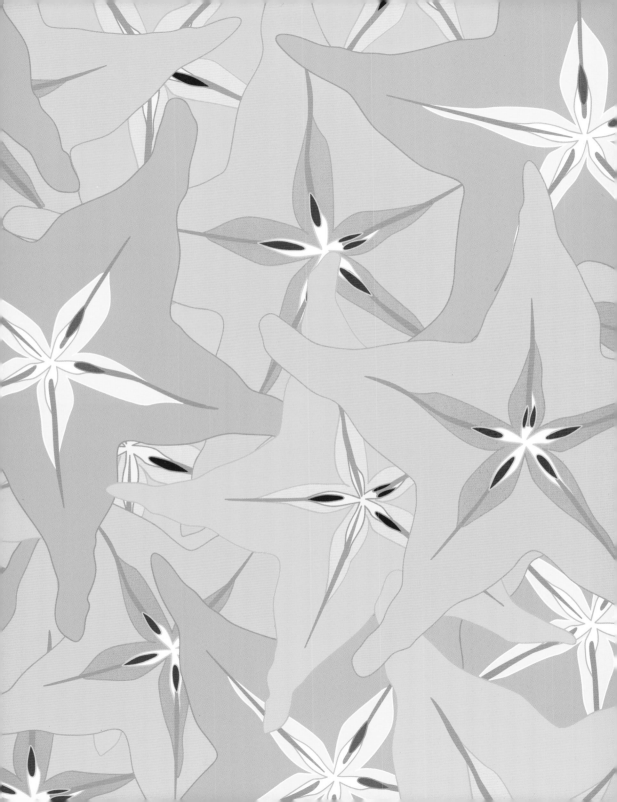

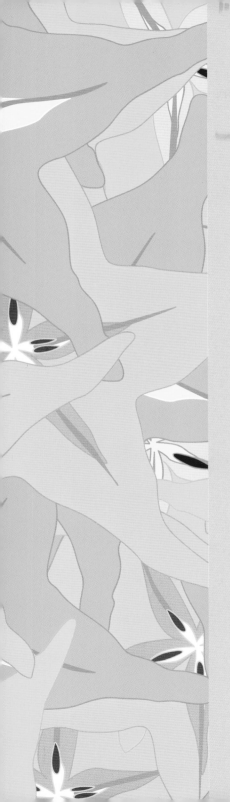

is for boosters

Now we come to the seriously **high-powered** juices. With a pure shot of energy, brimming with those **fabulous** nutrients that you need to keep your body fit and your brain sparking, plus our **targeted booster** ingredients. Visit your local health store and pick up the boost you need to **improve** your **performance**—spirulina to give you an intense nutrient boost, protein powder to build muscles, bee pollen to protect against the signs of aging. Choose the booster juices that will **benefit** you the most and give your juices a **nutrient boost.**

Grab them while you can

You know summer's really here when those juicy, ruby-red cherries get cheaper! Don't miss the opportunity to enjoy them when you can buy as many as you like.

cherry explosion

If you like cherries—those deep, dark bombs of flavor—you'll find they deliver energy in spades, and the coenzyme Q10 will keep you going all day.

3 apples, stemmed and quartered
½ banana
½ cup low-fat yogurt, frozen overnight,
   or low-fat yogurt plus 4 ice cubes
¾ cup cherries, pitted
1 teaspoon coenzyme Q10 powder

How to do it Put the apples through an electric juicer. (Alternatively, add ⅔ cup apple juice instead of juicing the apples.) Pour the juice into a blender or food processor, add all the remaining ingredients, including the coenzyme Q10 powder booster, and blend until smooth and creamy. Serve immediately.

NUTRIENTS:
Packed with: vitamins B2, B5, B6, B7, C; calcium, magnesium, manganese, phosphate, potassium, zinc; iodine
Plenty of: vitamins B1, B12, folic acid; copper
Also contains: vitamins B3, E, beta-carotene; iron; fiber; coenzyme Q10

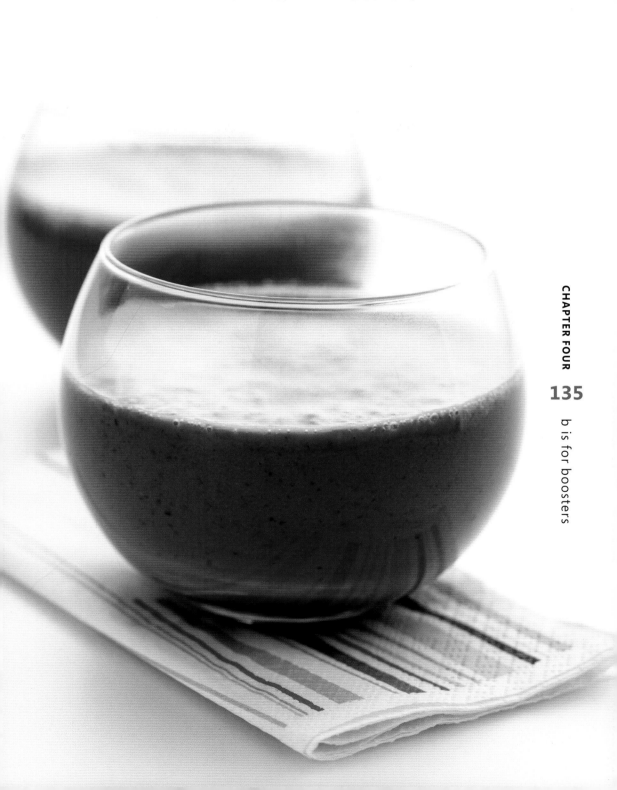

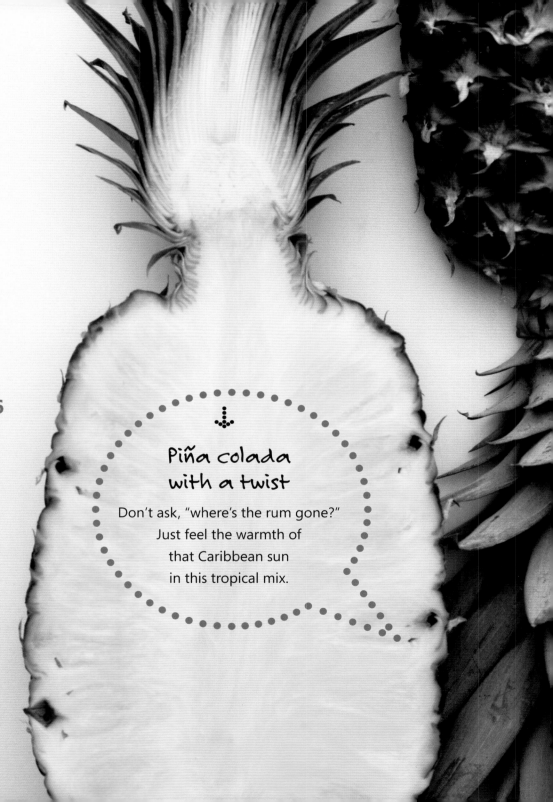

Piña colada
with a twist

Don't ask, "where's the rum gone?"
Just feel the warmth of
that Caribbean sun
in this tropical mix.

summer restore & revive

Need we say more? A smooth and creamy drink to soothe you through those hot summer days.

2 thin slices ginger root
2 pieces (about 2-inch cubes) peeled pineapple
⅔ cup soy milk
½ banana
½ cup soy yogurt, frozen overnight, or soy yogurt plus 4 ice cubes
¼ cup coconut milk
1 teaspoon ginseng powder

How to do it Put the ginger and pineapple through an electric juicer. Pour the juices into a blender or food processor, add all the remaining ingredients, including the ginseng powder booster, and blend until smooth and creamy. Serve immediately.

NUTRIENTS:
Packed with: vitamins B1, B2, B5, B6, B7, C; calcium, copper, magnesium, manganese, phosphate, potassium, zinc; iodine
Plenty of: vitamins B3, B12, beta-carotene, folic acid
Also contains: vitamin E; iron; fiber; isoflavones, omega-3, selenium

red, white & blue power smoothie

Feel young and energetic with this tofu and fruit combo that evens out hormone imbalances and fights those tell-tale signs of aging.

⅔ cup soy milk
½ banana
½ cup soy yogurt, frozen overnight, or soy yogurt plus 4 ice cubes
½ cup frozen blueberries
1¼ cups frozen raspberries
3 ounces silken tofu, cut into chunks
1 teaspoon chia seeds

How to do it Put all the ingredients, including the chia seed booster, in a blender or food processor and blend until smooth and creamy. Serve immediately.

NUTRIENTS:
Packed with: vitamins B1, B5, B6, B7, C, folic acid; calcium, copper, iron, magnesium, manganese, phosphate, potassium, zinc; fiber; iodine
Plenty of: vitamins B12, E, beta-carotene; selenium
Also contains: vitamin B3; ellagic acid, flavonoids, isoflavones

CHAPTER FOUR

berry breakfast

This breakfast granola pot is a real favorite—thick with oats, fruit and honey to make sure the most important meal of the day provides you with a healthy start.

⅔ cup soy milk
½ banana
½ cup soy yogurt, frozen overnight,
  or soy yogurt plus 4 ice cubes
¼ cup frozen blueberries
¼ cup frozen raspberries
1 teaspoon honey
½ cup granola
6 ice cubes
1 teaspoon wheat germ

✳ **How to make a booster smoothie**

   NUTRIENTS:
Packed with: vitamins B1, B2, B3, B5, B6, B7, B12, C, E, beta-carotene; calcium, copper, iron, magnesium, manganese, phosphate, potassium, zinc; fiber; iodine
Plenty of: folic acid
Also contains: ellagic acid, flavonoids; selenium

mango power buzz

When you need to be full of zing—performing at the top of your form—here's the juice that will give you maximum nutrient power.

⅔ cup soy milk
½ banana
½ cup soy yogurt, frozen overnight,
  or soy yogurt plus 4 ice cubes
1 mango, peeled and pitted
1¾ ounces silken tofu
6 tablespoons whey protein powder
1 teaspoon bee pollen granules

✳ **How to make a booster smoothie**

   NUTRIENTS:
Packed with: vitamins A, B1, B2, B3, B6, C, E, K, folic acid; calcium, potassium
Plenty of: omega-3, selenium
Also contains: magnesium

✳ **How to make a booster smoothie**
Put all the ingredients, including the wheat germ or whey protein powder and bee pollen boosters, in a blender or food processor and blend until smooth and creamy. Serve immediately.

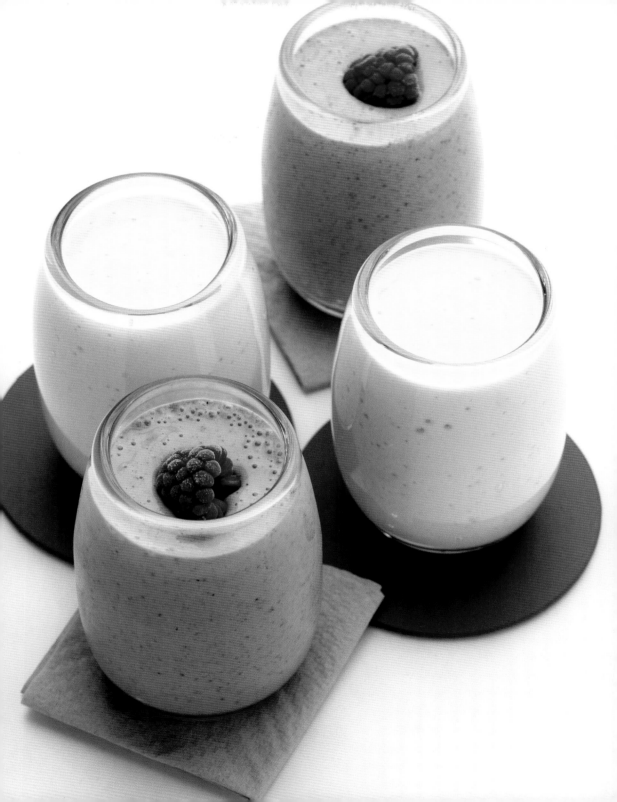

Ram-bam thank-you-ma'am!

Check out these wild-looking specimens. Slice round the skin, then peel off the lid to reveal the treasure inside.

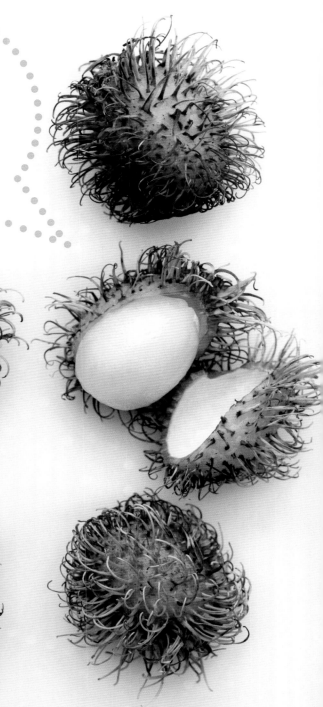

rambutan power

Buy your rambutans and coconut cubes from Asian stores to make this Thai-style smoothie with its creamy finish and delicate flavor. Use canned lychees if you cannot find rambutans.

½ pineapple, peeled and cut into chunks
½ banana
½ cup low-fat yogurt, frozen overnight, or low-fat yogurt plus 4 ice cubes
6 rambutans, peeled, pitted and frozen overnight
5½ ounces jarred or canned coconut gel cubes, drained
1 teaspoon l-glutamine

How to do it Put the pineapple through an electric juicer. (Alternatively, add ⅔ cup pineapple juice instead of juicing the pineapple.) Pour the juice into a blender or food processor, add all the remaining ingredients, including the l-glutamine booster, and blend until smooth and creamy. Serve immediately.

NUTRIENTS:
Packed with: vitamins B2, B5, B6, B7, C; calcium, manganese, phosphate, potassium; iodine
Plenty of: vitamins B1, B12, folic acid; magnesium, zinc;
Also contains: vitamins B3, E, beta-carotene; copper, iron; fiber; flavonoids; selenium

blueberry booster

A protein boost to take you through the afternoon with bright eyes and plenty of energy.

⅔ cup soy milk
½ banana
½ cup soy yogurt, frozen overnight, or soy yogurt plus 4 ice cubes
½ cup frozen blueberries
½ avocado, peeled and pitted
1 teaspoon protein powder

How to do it Put all the ingredients, including the protein powder booster, in a blender or food processor and blend until smooth and creamy. Serve immediately.

NUTRIENTS:
Packed with: vitamins B1, B2, B5, B6, B7, C; calcium, copper, magnesium, manganese, phosphate, potassium, zinc; fiber; iodine
Plenty of: vitamins B3, B12, beta-carotene, folic acid; iron; selenium
Also contains: vitamin E; ellagic acid, flavonoids, isoflavones

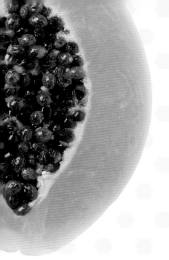

power enzymes

Enzymes are your body's nuclear reactors (or catalysts, to give them their proper name) that release energy from food. These are the guys that get digestion going. Your body produces its own digestive enzymes, but they are also present in raw foods—like the foods you use for juicing. Clever plant enzymes start breaking down your food before the enzymes you already have in your body kick in. Anything for an easy life.

Tell me more ...

When you break down the flesh of any fruit or vegetable—by chewing it, or by whizzing it in a juicer or blender—the enzymes become agitated and are ready to start extracting the goodness from the food in your stomach the minute they get there. They send vital nutrients out into your cells while your own digestive enzymes are still waking up to the fact that there's something to do. Yawn!

Ready for the science part? The four main groups of plant enzymes are: **proteases**, which break down proteins in your food; **amylases**, which turn complex sugars (polysaccharides) into something more pure and simple that your body can love; **lipases**, which get to work on the fats; and **cellulases**, which free up the fiber.

In the raw ...

If you want to commission your own army of enzymes for a body boot camp, then look no further than your own vegetable patch. And if you don't have one, then make sure you seek out the freshest fruits and vegetables at a store with a high turnover. They need to be totally fresh because enzymes are live, and they won't be active otherwise. And please clear out that veg drawer at the bottom of your fridge.

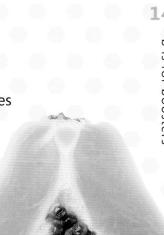

Easy does it!

Being healthy isn't rocket science
but it can seem like really hard work.
Rustling up a mung bean vegetable stew
is a bit of an effort.
Whizzing up a smoothie for
breakfast is just
so easy.

goji breakfast smoothie

You'll enjoy the mild, tangy flavor of goji berries, known for thousands of years to improve eyesight, boost the immune system and protect the liver.

⅔ cup soy milk
½ banana
½ cup soy yogurt, frozen overnight, or soy yogurt plus 4 ice cubes
1 teaspoon honey
⅓ cup granola
6 ice cubes
1 tablespoon goji berries

How to do it Put all the ingredients, including the goji berry booster, in a blender or food processor and blend until smooth and creamy. Serve immediately.

NUTRIENTS:
Packed with: vitamins B1, B2, B3, B5, B6, B7, C; calcium, copper, iron, magnesium, manganese, phosphate, potassium, zinc; fiber; iodine
Plenty of: vitamins B12, E, folic acid, beta-carotene
Also contains: isoflavones; selenium

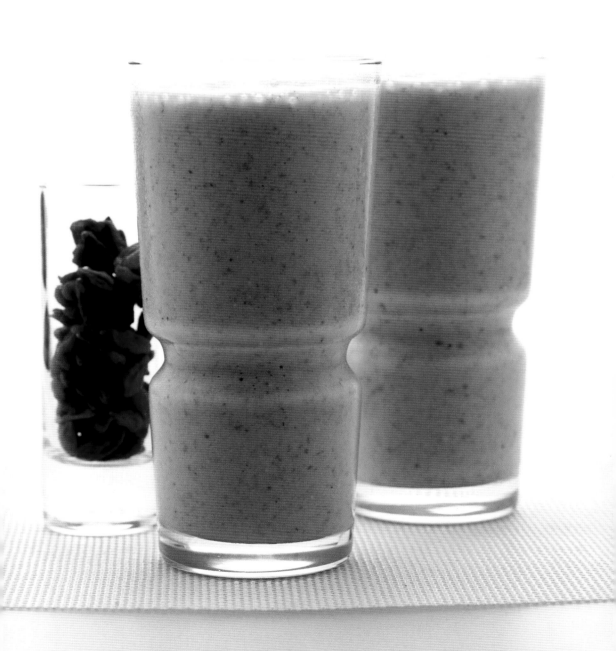

nature's mdma

Rich in vitamins and minerals, bee pollen brings us all the goodness of nature—highly concentrated. It's super-nourishment in a tiny package.

3 apples, stemmed and quartered
½ banana
½ cup low-fat yogurt, frozen overnight, or low-fat yogurt plus 4 ice cubes
2 pieces (about 2-inch cubes) peeled melon
2 dates, pitted
½ mango, peeled and pitted
1 apricot, pitted
1 teaspoon bee pollen granules

How to do it Put the apples through an electric juicer. (Alternatively, add ⅔ cup apple juice instead of juicing the apples.) Pour the juice into a blender or food processor, add all the remaining ingredients, including the bee pollen booster, and blend until smooth and creamy. Serve immediately.

> **NUTRIENTS:**
> **Packed with:** vitamins B1, B2, B3, B5, B6, B7, C, beta-carotene; calcium, copper, magnesium, manganese, phosphate, potassium; fiber; iodine
> **Plenty of:** vitamins B12, E, folic acid; iron, zinc
> **Also contains:** flavonoids

rich acai cherry

A small, round berry that is turned into a nutritious puree, acai adds healthy antioxidants to your system to help fight the signs of aging.

3 apples, stemmed and quartered
½ banana
½ cup low-fat yogurt, frozen overnight, or low-fat yogurt plus 4 ice cubes
15 cherries, pitted
1¾ ounces frozen acai puree
1 teaspoon agave syrup
1 teaspoon guarana seed powder

How to do it Put the apples through an electric juicer. (Alternatively, add ⅔ cup apple juice instead of juicing the apples.) Pour the juice into a blender or food processor, add all the remaining ingredients, including the guarana seed powder booster, and blend until smooth and creamy. Serve immediately.

> **NUTRIENTS:**
> **Packed with:** vitamins B1, B2, B5, B6, B7, C; calcium, iron, magnesium, phosphate, potassium; fiber; iodine
> **Plenty of:** vitamins B12, E, folic acid; manganese, zinc
> **Also contains:** vitamin B3, beta-carotene; copper; flavonoids

apricot tofu

Juicy and sweet should make you feel good enough, but the apricot's hidden secret is that it delivers chemicals that you can convert to serotonin. So there's a double whammy of the feel-good factor in this boosted smoothie.

⅔ cup soy milk
½ banana
½ cup soy yogurt, frozen overnight, or soy yogurt plus 4 ice cubes
2 apricots, pitted
1¾ ounces silken tofu, cut into chunks
1 teaspoon vitamin B5

How to do it Put all the ingredients, including the vitamin B5 booster, in a blender or food processor and blend until smooth and creamy. Serve immediately.

> **NUTRIENTS:**
> **Packed with:** vitamins B1, B2, B5, B6, B7, C, E, beta-carotene, folic acid; calcium, copper, magnesium, manganese, phosphate, potassium, zinc; iodine
> **Plenty of:** vitamins B3, B12; iron
> **Also contains:** fiber; flavonoids, isoflavones; selenium

peach & raspberry bunny

The perfect post-workout booster, peaches can help you overcome fatigue and ease those aching muscles. Brazilian guarana gives you an added boost of energy.

2 thin slices ginger root
3 oranges, halved
½ banana
½ cup low-fat yogurt, frozen overnight, or low-fat yogurt plus 4 ice cubes
½ peach, pitted
⅓ cup frozen raspberries
1 teaspoon guarana seed powder

How to do it Put the ginger through an electric juicer. Squeeze the juice from the oranges. Pour the juices into a blender or food processor, add all the remaining ingredients, including the guarana seed powder booster, and blend until smooth and creamy. Serve immediately.

> **NUTRIENTS:**
> **Packed with:** vitamins B2, B5, B6, B7, C, beta-carotene, folic acid; calcium, magnesium, phosphate, potassium; iodine
> **Plenty of:** vitamins B1, B3, B12; copper, iron, manganese, zinc; fiber
> **Also contains:** vitamin E; ellagic acid, flavonoids

The magic of manuka

When your throat is sore and your nose feels blocked, try our remedy for that winter cold that combines the soothing qualities of manuka honey with the power of echinacea.

winter cold buster

If you suffer from winter colds, it can make you really miserable—runny nose, itchy eyes, sore throat. This immune-system boost helps send those germs packing.

3 thin slices ginger root
5 oranges, halved
½ lime
15 drops echinacea
1 teaspoon manuka honey

How to do it Put the ginger through an electric juicer. Squeeze the juice from the oranges and the lime. Stir the juices together with the echinacea and manuka honey boosters and serve immediately.

NUTRIENTS:
Packed with: vitamins A, C, folic acid; calcium, iron, magnesium, phosphate, potassium
Plenty of: vitamins B1, B2, B3, B6; calcium

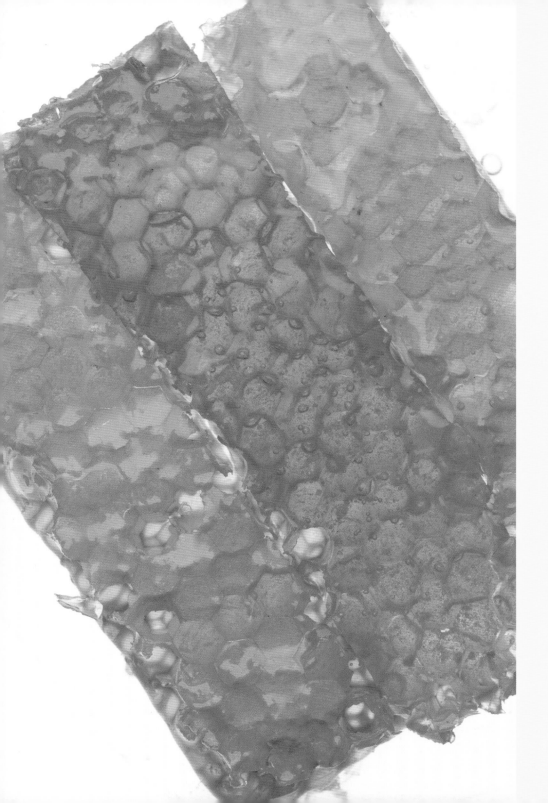

Forgot to stretch?

Aching muscles?
One too many circuits?
We have a juicing solution.
This is the perfect wind-
down soother.

cherri-licious

If you've overdone the exercise and your joints and muscles are aching, choose a juice with plenty of pineapple to reduce the inflammation—especially when it contains cherries with their own anti-inflammatory properties.

¼ pineapple, peeled and cut into chunks
½ banana
½ cup low-fat yogurt, frozen overnight, or low-fat yogurt plus 4 ice cubes
⅓ cup cherries, pitted
1 tablespoon aloe vera juice

NUTRIENTS:
Packed with: vitamins B1, B2, B5, B6, B7, C; calcium, magnesium, manganese, phosphate, potassium, zinc; iodine
Plenty of: vitamin B12, beta-carotene, folic acid; copper
Also contains: vitamins E, B3; iron; fiber

How to do it Put the pineapple through an electric juicer. (Alternatively, add ⅔ cup pineapple juice instead of juicing the pineapple.) Pour the juice into a blender or food processor, add all the remaining ingredients, including the aloe vera juice booster, and blend until smooth and creamy. Serve immediately.

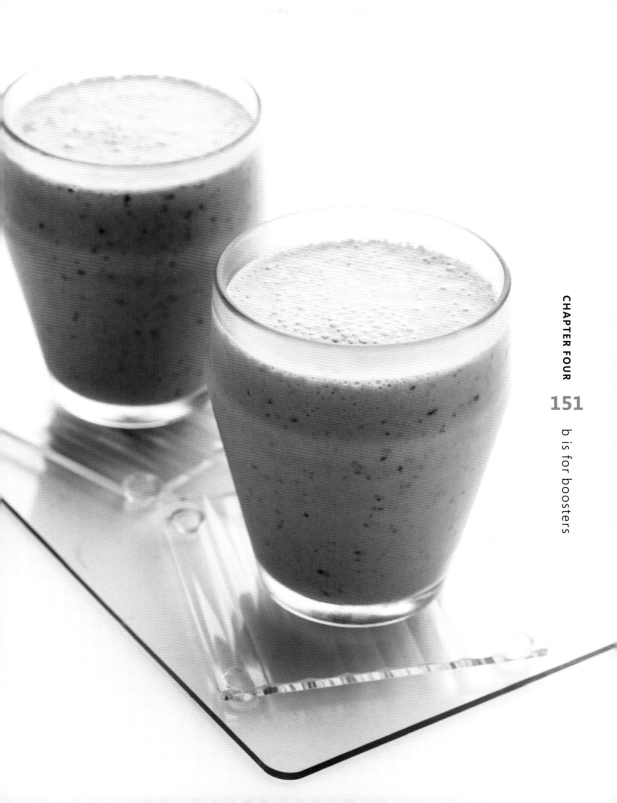

jump
with fitness

Ultimate fitness requires a combination of physical strength, optimum health and a focused mind. Any athlete will tell you that a fresh juice can pack strength, power and energy. You may have your sights on being an Olympian; or more likely you just want to tone up, be strong and chill out. No time for a gym session? Virtually fat-free, but jumping with fiber, vitamins and healthy carbs, fitness juices are one step on the path to the body and mind you always dreamed of.

Why is that?

Fitness is more than just about having energy and staying slim and strong. It's also about having the mental capacity to cope with the everyday demands life throws at you. Over the course of one day, you can provide your body with nutrients that give you back the strength to grab life, live it and love it.

So what does your body need to be its personal best? **Vitamin A** keeps you bright-eyed and bushy-tailed, and gives you eyes that shine. **Vitamin C** fires up your immune system. **Iron** supplies you with energy—and what is fitness without energy? **Lignans** help keep your heart healthy. **Manganese** provides bone power, pure and simple. **Potassium** is the cheapest health insurance you can buy, protecting your heart and mind from stress.

Where do we get all that?

Follow the fitness-juice rainbow—with every color comes a host of different nutrients. Create juices using foods in each color group and take a leap to your peak.

RED—beets, cherries, lychees, raspberries, redcurrants, strawberries.

YELLOW—bananas, grapefruit, pineapples.

> **ORANGE**—apricots, cantaloupe melons, mangoes, oranges, papayas, peaches.

> **GREEN**—broccoli, cucumbers, kale, spinach.

> **PURPLE**—blueberries, prunes.

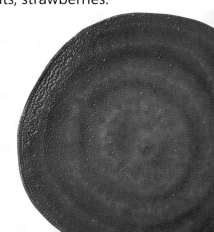

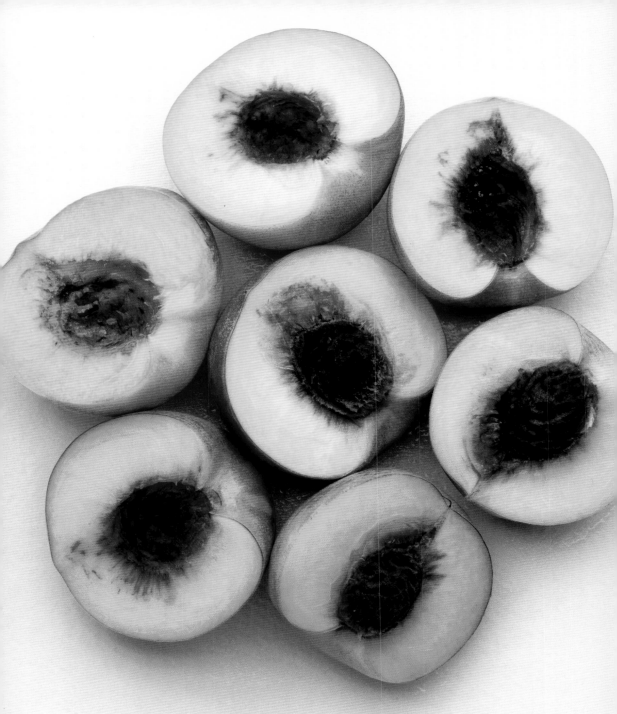

Yoga buffs look no further

peach performance

We created this recipe for the sexy, slim yoga or pilates buff! Peach is great for muscle recovery and is a renowned performance enhancer and energizer. Add the softness of the tofu and it makes a perfect after-session smoothie.

⅔ cup soy milk
½ banana
½ cup soy yogurt, frozen overnight, or soy yogurt plus 4 ice cubes
1 peach, pitted
½ passionfruit, seeds scooped out
5½ ounces silken tofu, cut into chunks
1 teaspoon ginseng powder

How to do it Put all the ingredients, including the ginseng powder booster, in a blender or food processor and blend until smooth and creamy. Serve immediately.

NUTRIENTS:
Packed with: vitamins B1, B2, B5, B6, B7, C, beta-carotene; calcium, copper, magnesium, manganese, phosphate, potassium, zinc; iodine,
Plenty of: vitamins B3, B12, folic acid; iron; selenium
Also contains: vitamin E; fiber; ginseng, isoflavones

vitamin boost

An array of vitamins is waiting in this glass, with a special blast of B, C and beta-carotene. Add a handful of strawberries if you don't have guava.

5 apples, stemmed and quartered
½ guava, peeled
1 kiwi, peeled and halved
10 canned lychees, frozen overnight
1 teaspoon vitamin C powder

How to do it Put the apples and guava through an electric juicer. Pour the juices into a blender or food processor, add the remaining ingredients, including the vitamin C powder booster, and blend until smooth. Serve immediately.

NUTRIENTS:
Packed with: vitamins C, beta-carotene; calcium, copper, phosphate
Plenty of: vitamin B6; magnesium, potassium; fiber
Also contains: vitamins B1, B2, B3, B5, B7; iron, manganese, zinc; flavonoids

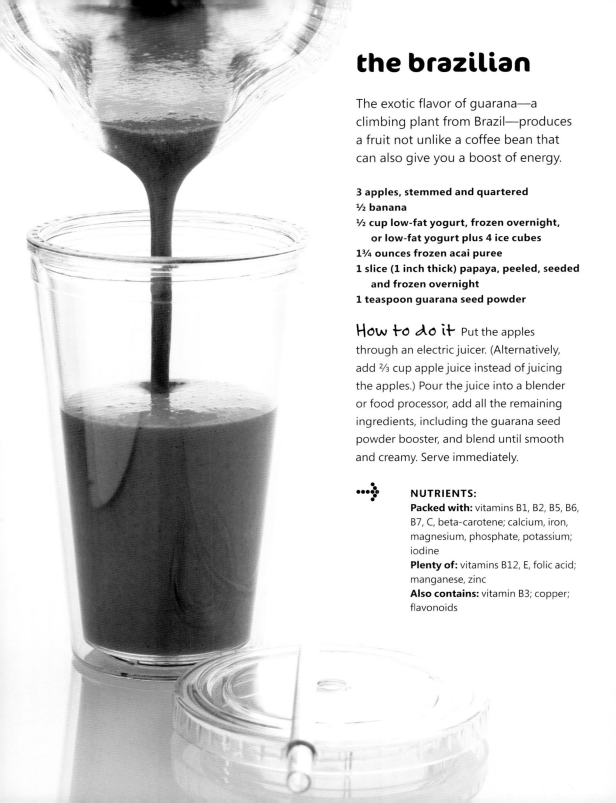

the brazilian

The exotic flavor of guarana—a climbing plant from Brazil—produces a fruit not unlike a coffee bean that can also give you a boost of energy.

3 apples, stemmed and quartered
½ banana
½ cup low-fat yogurt, frozen overnight,
  or low-fat yogurt plus 4 ice cubes
1¾ ounces frozen acai puree
1 slice (1 inch thick) papaya, peeled, seeded
  and frozen overnight
1 teaspoon guarana seed powder

How to do it Put the apples through an electric juicer. (Alternatively, add ⅔ cup apple juice instead of juicing the apples.) Pour the juice into a blender or food processor, add all the remaining ingredients, including the guarana seed powder booster, and blend until smooth and creamy. Serve immediately.

NUTRIENTS:
Packed with: vitamins B1, B2, B5, B6, B7, C, beta-carotene; calcium, iron, magnesium, phosphate, potassium; iodine
Plenty of: vitamins B12, E, folic acid; manganese, zinc
Also contains: vitamin B3; copper; flavonoids

super-flex joints

We all want to stay supple, and this combination of nutrients will help you keep your joints flexible. Just add gentle exercise!

⅔ cup soy milk
½ banana
½ cup soy yogurt, frozen overnight, or soy yogurt plus 4 ice cubes
½ avocado, peeled and pitted
½ mango, peeled and pitted
2 pieces (about 2-inch cubes) peeled melon
½ cup rolled oats
1 tablespoon sunflower seeds
1 teaspoon omega oil

How to do it Put all the ingredients, including the omega oil booster, in a blender or food processor and blend until smooth and creamy. Serve immediately.

NUTRIENTS:
Packed with: vitamins B1, B2, B3, B5, B6, B7, C, E, beta-carotene, folic acid; calcium, copper, iron, magnesium, manganese, phosphate, potassium, zinc; fiber; iodine
Plenty of: vitamin B12
Also contains: isoflavones, selenium

starfruit healer

Here is a vitamin C bonanza to improve your immunity, protect against circulatory problems—and taste great! Pineapple or mango would work instead of the starfruit.

1½ starfruit, cut into chunks
5 apples, stemmed and quartered
2 tablespoons aloe vera juice

How to do it Put the starfruit and apples through an electric juicer. Stir the juices together with the aloe vera juice booster and serve immediately.

NUTRIENTS:
Packed with: vitamin C
Plenty of: potassium
Also contains: vitamins B1, B2, B3, B5, B6, B7, folic acid; calcium, iron, magnesium, phosphate; fiber; flavonoids

Time for
a guarana break

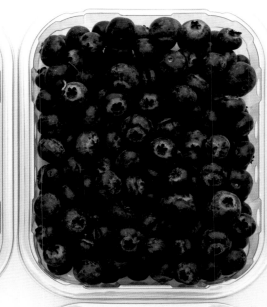

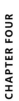

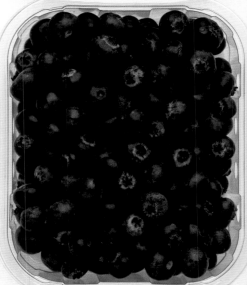

Superfood this way

Tiny but intense.
Blueberries are
power-packed
with antioxidants.

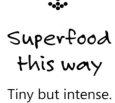

kickstart super smoothie

Start the day with a kick of energy, or give yourself a boost when you hit that mid-afternoon slump. This smoothie is good to stimulate the gray cells and liven up the body.

3 oranges, halved
½ banana
½ cup low-fat yogurt, frozen overnight,
**   or low-fat yogurt plus 4 ice cubes**
¼ cup frozen blueberries
¾ cup frozen raspberries
½ mango, peeled and pitted
1 teaspoon vitamin C powder

How to do it Squeeze the juice from the oranges. (Alternatively, add ⅔ cup orange juice instead of squeezing the oranges.) Pour the juice into a blender or food processor, add all the remaining ingredients, including the vitamin C powder booster, and blend until smooth and creamy. Serve immediately.

NUTRIENTS:
Packed with: vitamins B1, B2, B5, B6, B7, C, beta-carotene; calcium, copper, magnesium, manganese, phosphate, potassium; fiber; iodine
Plenty of: vitamins B3, B12, E, folic acid; iron, zinc
Also contains: ellagic acid, flavonoids

mmo with ginseng

Three of our favorite ingredients make this sunny, bright booster, packed with antioxidants to keep you looking and feeling young.

5 oranges, halved
2 pieces (about 2-inch cubes) peeled melon
½ mango, peeled and pitted
1 teaspoon ginseng powder

How to do it Squeeze the juice from the oranges. (Alternatively, add ⅔ cup orange juice instead of squeezing the oranges.) Pour the juice into a blender or food processor, add all the remaining ingredients, including the ginseng powder booster, and blend until smooth and creamy. Serve immediately.

NUTRIENTS:
Packed with: vitamins B6, C, beta-carotene; potassium, magnesium, manganese
Plenty of: vitamins B1, B3, folic acid; copper, iron, phosphate; fiber
Also contains: vitamins B2, B5, B7, E; calcium, zinc; flavonoids

fat burner

With the rich supply of nutrients in this red and purple berry combo, you'll feel fuller and less inclined to snack, helping you keep control of your weight.

••••⑅

3 apples, stemmed and quartered
½ banana
½ cup low-fat yogurt, frozen overnight,
    or low-fat yogurt plus 4 ice cubes
¼ cup frozen blueberries
5 frozen strawberries
¼ cup frozen cranberries
¼ cup frozen raspberries
1 teaspoon fat burner booster

How to do it Put the apples through an electric juicer. (Alternatively, add ⅔ cup apple juice instead of juicing the apples.) Pour the juices into a blender or food processor, add all the remaining ingredients, including the fat burner booster, and blend until smooth and creamy. Serve immediately.

NUTRIENTS:
Packed with: vitamins B2, B5, B6, B7, C, beta-carotene; calcium, copper, magnesium, manganese, phosphate, potassium, zinc; fiber; iodine
Plenty of: vitamins B1, B12, folic acid; iron
Also contains: vitamins B3, E; ellagic acid, flavonoids

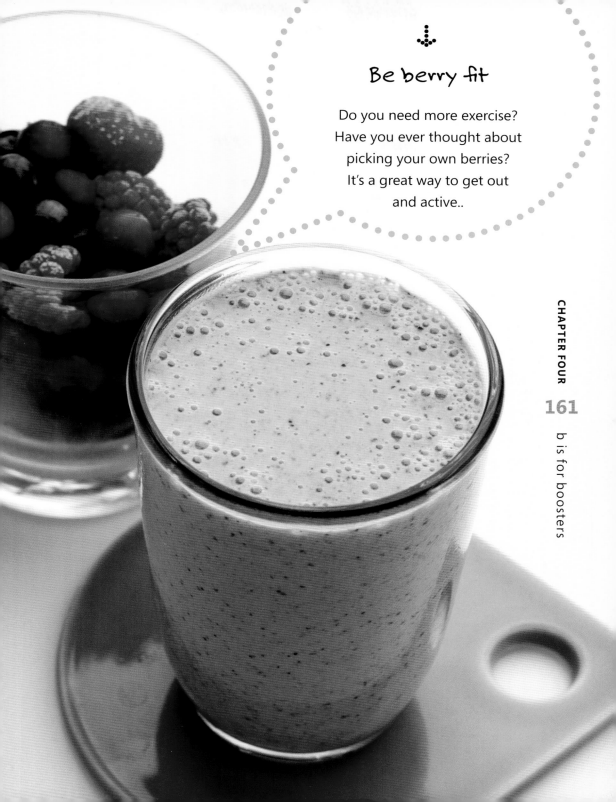

Be berry fit

Do you need more exercise?
Have you ever thought about
picking your own berries?
It's a great way to get out
and active..

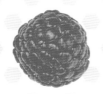

burst berries

From al fresco picnics to forest rambles, berries are the stuff of childhood memories, always numbered among our favorite teatime treats and baked into the tastiest desserts. Red, purple, blue, the deep colors found in berry juices tell you that every sip is bursting with goodness. When it comes to berries, good things really do come in small packages.

Why is that?

All berries practically ooze antioxidants (particularly vitamins C and E) and phenols, are high in fiber and have a low glycemic index. They are low in calories, too. (And therefore clearly a gift from the gods!) You don't even have to wait for them to come into season—berries freeze beautifully, keeping all their delicious goodness, so stock up for the year and juice away.

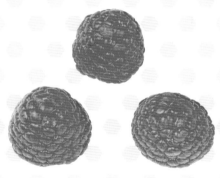

What will berries do for me?

- **Make your eyes sparkle**—raspberries and blueberries contain lutein, an antioxidant that protects the cells of the eyes. (And the skin, too, to keep it smooth and supple.)

- **Give you luscious locks**—strawberries contain high levels of folic acid, wonderful for strong, beautiful hair. Cranberries, blueberries and blackberries keep it shiny.

- **Fight, fight, fight**—an army of antioxidants is ready to help prevent damage to your precious cells. When it comes to disease, berries mean war.

- **Keep you powerful**—many berries, but especially blueberries, contain heart-protective anthocyanins in their skins.

Figs were the food of
the first Olympians

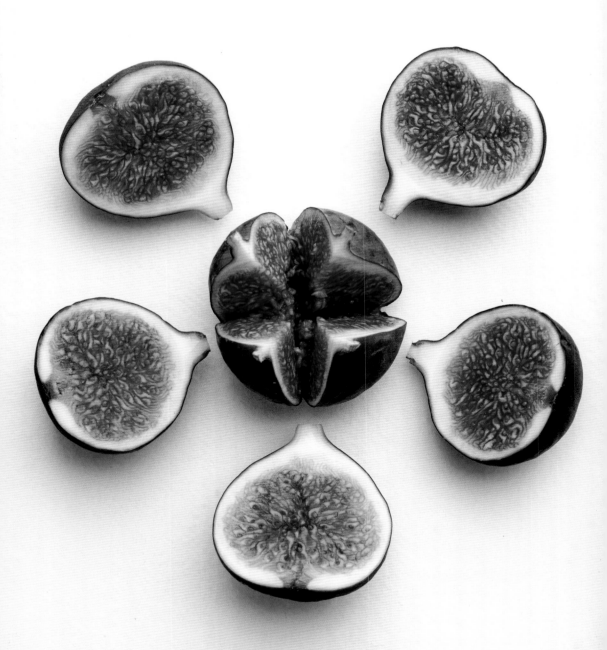

green earth

Spirulina contains a greater concentration of nutrients than any other food, so it packs a real punch in the health stakes. Try maple syrup instead of agave, too.

3 apples, stemmed and quartered
½ banana
½ cup low-fat yogurt, frozen overnight, or low-fat yogurt plus 4 ice cubes
1 tablespoon cacao nibs
3 figs
1 tablespoon walnuts
½ cup granola
1 teaspoon agave syrup
1 teaspoon spirulina powder

How to do it Put the apples through an electric juicer. (Alternatively, add ⅔ cup apple juice instead of juicing the apples.) Pour the juice into a blender or food processor, add all the remaining ingredients, including the spirulina powder booster, and blend until smooth and creamy. Serve immediately.

NUTRIENTS:
Packed with: vitamins B1, B2, B3, B5, B6, B7, C, folic acid; calcium, copper, iron, magnesium, manganese, phosphate, potassium, zinc; fiber; iodine
Plenty of: vitamins B12, E, beta-carotene
Also contains: flavonoids

banana, date & walnut

Chia seeds are the new super-booster—promoting a healthy heart and stabilizing blood sugar levels—making this a real lunchtime bonus.

3 apples, stemmed and quartered
½ banana
½ cup low-fat yogurt, frozen overnight, or low-fat yogurt plus 4 ice cubes
¾ cup dates, pitted
1 tablespoon walnuts
1 teaspoon agave syrup
1 teaspoon chia seeds

How to do it Put the apples through an electric juicer. (Alternatively, add ⅔ cup apple juice instead of juicing the apples.) Pour the juice into a blender or food processor, add all the remaining ingredients, including the chia seed booster, and blend until smooth and creamy. Serve immediately.

NUTRIENTS:
Packed with: vitamins B1, B2, B5, B6, B7, C; calcium, copper, magnesium, manganese, phosphate, potassium, zinc; iodine
Plenty of: vitamins B3, B12, beta-carotene, folic acid; iron; fiber
Also contains: vitamin E; flavonoids

copacabana super stamina

We may not all be able to go to Rio but we can all imagine lazing in the sun on that fabulous beach. And what better way to stimulate the imagination than this smoothie.

⅔ cup soy milk
½ banana
½ cup soy yogurt, frozen overnight, or soy yogurt plus 4 ice cubes
½ cup cherries, pitted
1¾ ounces frozen acai puree
1 teaspoon ginseng powder

How to do it Put all the ingredients, including the ginseng powder booster, in a blender or food processor and blend until smooth and creamy. Serve immediately.

NUTRIENTS:
Packed with: vitamins A, C; copper, manganese, potassium, zinc; flavonoids
Plenty of: vitamins, B1, B2, B3, folic acid; iron, magnesium, phosphate
Also contains: calcium, selenium

gingered roots & spirulina

Packed with essential amino acids, spirulina is a complete protein and a great source of B vitamins, so it's especially useful for vegetarians. It is derived from kelp and available in powdered form.

1 beet, cut into chunks
2 thin slices ginger root
8 carrots, tops removed
1 teaspoon spirulina powder

How to do it Put the beet, ginger and carrots through an electric juicer. Stir the juices together with the spirulina powder booster and serve immediately.

NUTRIENTS:
Packed with: vitamins B1, B6, C, beta-carotene, folic acid; copper, magnesium, manganese, phosphate, potassium
Plenty of: vitamins B5, E; calcium, iron, zinc,
Also contains: vitamins B2, B3, B7; flavonoids, omega-3

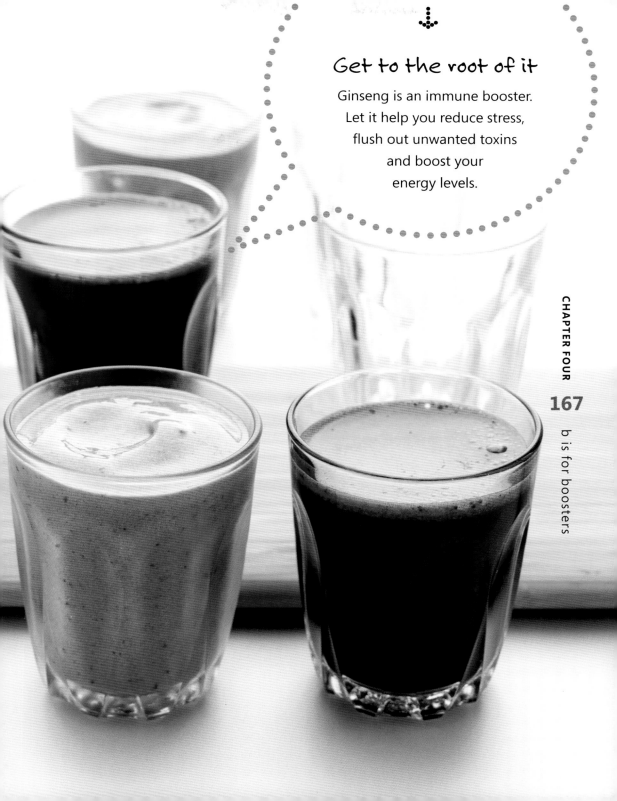

Get to the root of it

Ginseng is an immune booster.
Let it help you reduce stress,
flush out unwanted toxins
and boost your
energy levels.

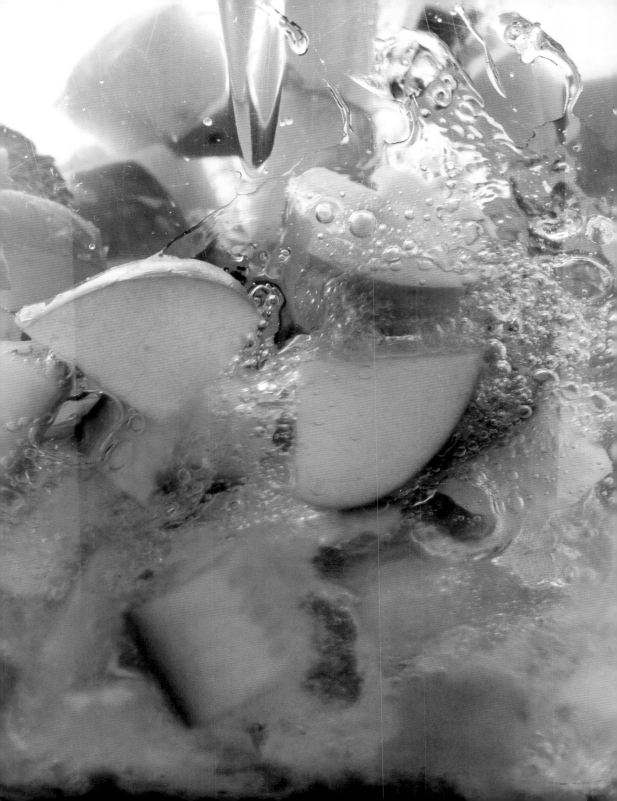

aloe appetizer

Soothing is the name of the game. Let this slide through your system, calming and restoring all the way.

3 apples, stemmed and quartered
1 apple, stemmed, peeled, cored and frozen overnight
¼ cucumber
3 mint leaves
1 teaspoon aloe vera juice

How to do it Put the unfrozen apples through an electric juicer. (Alternatively, add ⅔ cup apple juice instead of juicing the apples.) Pour the juice into a blender or food processor, add all the remaining ingredients, including the aloe vera juice booster, and blend until smooth and creamy. Serve immediately.

NUTRIENTS:
Packed with: vitamins A, C, K; calcium, potassium
Plenty of: iron, magnesium, manganese
Also contains: vitamins B1, B2, B6

hay fever buster

When summer arrives and the pollen is in the air, don't let it get you down. Enlist the help of the humble bee and some hedgerow favorites. A spoonful of local honey a day will help build up your immunity.

5 oranges, halved
½ cup blackberries
¼ cup blackcurrants
1 teaspoon bee pollen granules
1 teaspoon local honey

How to do it Squeeze the juice from the oranges. (Alternatively, add ⅔ cup orange juice instead of squeezing the oranges.) Pour the juice into a blender or food processor, add all the remaining ingredients, including the bee pollen granule booster, and blend until smooth and creamy. Serve immediately.

NUTRIENTS:
Packed with: vitamins B1, B6, C, beta-carotene, folic acid; copper, magnesium, manganese, phosphate, potassium
Plenty of: vitamins B5, E; calcium, iron, zinc
Also contains: vitamins B2, B3, B7; flavonoids, omega-3

Bee pollen tip:
start taking it six weeks
before hay fever
season begins

red & ginger

To purify the blood, give you energy and protect from diseases, here's the drink favored by Olympians to build their strength and energy. It'll certainly keep you on your toes.

1 beet, cut into chunks
2 thin slices ginger root
1 handful of parsley leaves
8 carrots, tops removed
2 tablespoons aloe vera juice

How to do it Put all the ingredients, except the aloe vera juice booster, through an electric juicer. Stir the juices together with the aloe vera juice booster and serve immediately.

NUTRIENTS:
Packed with: vitamins B1, B5, B6, C, beta-carotene, folic acid; copper, iron, magnesium, manganese, phosphate, potassium
Plenty of: vitamin E; calcium, zinc
Also contains: vitamins B2, B3, B7, K; flavonoids, omega-3

cool, calm, collected

Relax and go with the flow. This booster smoothie is perfect to help you keep your composure, maintain your brain function and stay on top of everything. You could also use almond milk (see page 129) instead of soy milk, if you like.

1 pear, stemmed and quartered
¼ cucumber
⅔ cup soy milk
½ banana
½ cup soy yogurt, frozen overnight, or soy yogurt plus 4 ice cubes
1 slice (1 inch thick) papaya, peeled, seeded and frozen overnight
1 teaspoon ginkgo biloba

How to do it Put the pear and cucumber through an electric juicer. Pour the juices into a blender or food processor, add all the remaining ingredients, including the ginkgo biloba booster, and blend until smooth and creamy. Serve immediately.

NUTRIENTS:
Packed with: vitamins B1, B2, B5, B6, B7, C, folic acid; calcium, copper, magnesium, phosphate, potassium; fiber
Plenty of: vitamins B3, B12, beta-carotene; iron, manganese, zinc; iodine
Also contains: vitamin E; selenium

summer flu fighter

Everyone hates summer colds, so ward them off with a dose of veggies to boost the immune system and help make sure your summer is sneeze-free.

½ watermelon, peeled, seeded and cut
    into chunks
¼ fennel bulb
1 handful of parsley leaves
½ mango, peeled and pitted
10 drops echinacea

How to do it Put the watermelon, fennel and parsley through an electric juicer. Pour the juices into a blender or food processor, add the remaining ingredients, including the echinacea booster, and blend until smooth and creamy. Serve immediately.

NUTRIENTS:
Packed with: vitamins B1, B5, B6, C, beta-carotene, folic acid; copper, iron, magnesium, manganese, potassium
Plenty of: vitamins B3, B7, E, K; calcium, phosphate, zinc; fiber
Also contains: vitamin B2

pappy cress

Stimulating and cleansing, the peppery taste of watercress flavors this booster and hints at its ability to purify the blood, making your liver function effectively—with the added bonus of a glow to the skin.

1 papaya, peeled, seeded and cut into
    chunks
2 handfuls of watercress
3 apples, stemmed and quartered
½ lime
1 teaspoon vitamin C powder

How to do it Put the papaya, watercress and apples through an electric juicer. Stir the juices together, squeeze in the lime juice and add the vitamin C powder booster. Serve immediately.

NUTRIENTS:
Packed with: vitamins B1, C, beta-carotene; copper, iron, magnesium, manganese, phosphate, potassium; fiber
Plenty of: vitamin B2, B5, B6; calcium
Also contains: vitamins B3, B7, E, K, folic acid; zinc; limonene

Spell-binding stuff

Pumpkin is a real high-flyer in the nutrient stakes. Juice the flesh and seeds and you'll be scoring for your home team.

liquid luck

You don't need to be a wizard to see the magic in this boosted juice with nutrients that make the whole body sparkle.

2 pieces (about 2-inch cubes) pumpkin, peeled
3 oranges, halved
¼ lime
½ banana
½ cup low-fat yogurt, frozen overnight, or low-fat yogurt plus 4 ice cubes
seeds from 3 cardamom pods
1 teaspoon pumpkin seeds
1 teaspoon chia seeds

NUTRIENTS:
Packed with: vitamins B1, B2, B5, B6, B7, C, beta-carotene; calcium, magnesium, manganese, phosphate, potassium; iodine
Plenty of: vitamins B12, E, folic acid; iron, zinc
Also contains: vitamin B3; copper; fiber; flavonoids

How to do it Put the pumpkin in a steamer over a pan of boiling water, cover and cook about 8 minutes until tender. Leave to cool. Squeeze the juice from the oranges and lime. Pour the juices into a blender or food processor, add all the remaining ingredients, including the pumpkin and the chia seed boosters, and blend until smooth and creamy. Serve immediately.

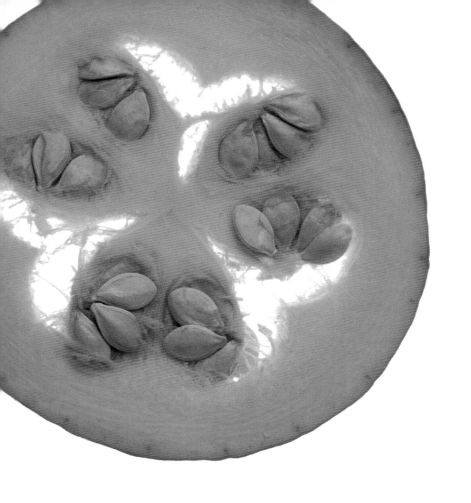
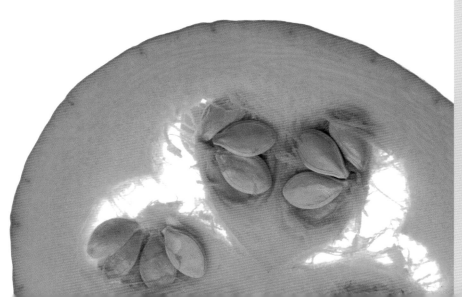

index

174

e is for energy, f is for fig, g is for guava, h is for honey,

Acknowledgments

My thanks to all at DBP for their support and advice with our first-ever Crussh book, especially Grace, Manisha, Wendy and Sailesh, who helped nudge us through as we ran up against publishing deadlines!

Special thanks to Tom, Catia, Ilva, Gil and Daniella, Imma, Winston, Kasia and the Cornhill team, Laura and Arran, Ewa and Marzenna and the HSK team, and Magda for contributing fantastic recipes.

Also thanks to Nick, Yvonne, Sylvie; José, Henry and the Rathbone team; Imma and the BBC team for being hugely helpful in making, tasting and testing our recipes!

Picture Credits

All photography by *William Lingwood* except for those listed below:

Chris Fung:
    P. 4.

Nicolas Raymond/Shutterstock:
    P. 162–3.

Simon Smith:
    P. 42–3, 58–9, 68–9, 96–7, 110–11, 120–21, 142–3, 152–3.

I is for index

THE END